MW01532198

Twenty-five days

Will Jelbert

Copyright © 2016 by Will Jelbert
All rights reserved. This book or any portion thereof may not be reproduced or
used in any manner without the express written permission of the author.
ISBN-13: 978-1530167074 ISBN-10: 1530167078
Cover design by Dil2014

For Happiness Coaching, Corporate and Personal Communications
Coaching, & Personal Training for Happiness visit:
www.happinessanimal.com or email the author:
w@happinessanimal.com

For Gina

<u>Contents</u>

<u>Introduction</u>

If I captured all the thoughts I had between the night at the restaurant when I first met my future fiancée and submitting the online divorce application, I could map out a chain of thinking links, associated actions and attractions that led from fried chicken, not only to marriage, but also to divorce. One Christmas holiday I drove my four-wheel-drive from Sydney to Brisbane doing as much of the journey off-road as possible. Somewhere along the way, following a dirt track, my ex-wife and I found ourselves lost in an Australian rainforest. I didn't know it at the time, but this turned out to be a critical turning point in my life. I realized I was lost in the rainforest and in my marriage because I had no idea how I came to be there in the first place. I was not using one vital connection to happiness, namely awareness, and the other four muscles that would have enabled me to connect well with my existence were in atrophy. Following this 'lost in the rainforest moment' I had a near-fatal accident. After a year of recovery and follow up surgeries to reconstruct my face, and a divorce, I was determined to make sense of how I had got to the rainforest in the first place and if the marriage, the money, the apartment, the restaurants and the rainforest weren't going to make me happy, then what would?

To answer that question, I began four years of research for my first book, *The Happiness Animal*. I supported my own studies with the core ideas of the world's most respected psychologists in the field of happiness, each bringing their own specialist expertise. My approach to writing *The Happiness Animal* was to create the only book anyone (myself included) would ever need to exercise happiness. What I quickly discovered when I introduced the exercises – first to those I knew, then to my happiness training clients, and to the tens of thousands of readers around the world - is that what makes people happy is universal. I know the exercises I gave readers in *The Happiness Animal* work because I have used them with my coaching clients in the USA, Europe and Australia with great success. But I realize now that I'd been so focused on my clients, on happiness theory, and on completing *The Happiness Animal* that I'd forgotten to write about my own experience of getting happier. That's where this book comes in. It's my story of taking one happiness exercise a day, and diarizing how I feel before, during and after each exercise. I hope you enjoy this journey with me. If you do, you can start your own journey at the end of this book where I have provided instructions for all the exercises I use...

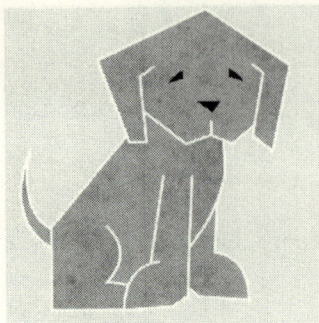

__Chapter 1__

Five days honest

Telling the truth is like an exercise and diet program that works to improve your strength and resistance over a period of time

Brad Blanton

That which is false troubles the heart, but truth brings joyous tranquility

Rumi

Pride prefers a mask to her own face

Seneca

Day 1: 'Be sincere with me dear' (exercising sincerity)

I got out of bed at least an hour earlier than normal this Wednesday morning. My French friend Jacques is visiting me and we've already been for a long walk from the farm to the river through the Australian bush and back. It's after lunch and I'm sitting on the deck at the corner of the house overlooking the small lake at the farm I'm house sitting near Canberra, Australia. The sun is shining, the birds chirping. I'm feeling the post-lunch drop in energy and staying awake feels like a small effort. Jacques is asleep on the sofa in front of the fire. I've already done my work for the day and applied for some jobs in New York. I'm sleepy, sitting comfortably, surrounded by birdsong, crickets and the occasional bird splashing into the lake.

The first part of the exercise is done alone, with a piece of text. The piece of text I've decided to use is taken from the book I'm currently reading, *Thinking Fast and Slow* by Daniel Kahnemann. I start taking one short phrase and repeating it three times before moving onto the next phrase. I notice that the more I repeat a phrase, the more I begin to visualize each word. Strangely enough, the more phrases I repeat, connecting with a visual of each word in each phrase, the less tired I feel. Mid-way through the paragraph I start to feel a sense of heightened awareness of my senses: Light seems brighter, colors more noticeable, and I feel instantly present. I'm not thinking thoughts about anything that I can't see or hear right here right now. Immediate focus. No distraction. Clarity. My breathing slows. I focus on each word. Then I catch myself smiling and laughing. Tension from tiredness around my eyes, forehead, crown, it seems to evaporate. I feel more at ease and relaxed, yet awake. It's a sense of cognitive ease and alertness in one. When I read the word 'feeling' aloud, I feel a tingle down my spine. I continue reading and repeating the short phrases, three times each for about 10 minutes, until I feel fully energized and relaxed.

Next, I open the sliding glass doors on the deck and go inside. My friend Jacques wakes up and asks me if I want to do the exercise (which I have briefed him on earlier today). I say yes. Jacques sits on the couch and I pull up a dining-room chair opposite him. I show him the text I am going to read to him and ask him to interrupt and ask me to clarify any of the points he doesn't get a clear picture of as I read the words. In response to his questions, I am only allowed to clarify by repeating words that I have already used.

I begin reading. For the first few phrases, Jacques interrupts me and asks me to repeat. I notice with these phrases I am more self-conscious, worried about embarrassing myself or not being able to perform as a reader in front of my friend. But the more I read, the more I start to visualize each word again, as I had done with the solo part of the exercise. I notice Jacques eyes are sparkling with light. I again feel more focused, with no thoughts, and it's an almost meditative clearness of head.

Once I finish reading the paragraph to Jacques, he gives me some feedback on how he felt during the exercise. Here are some of the comments:

'You seemed completely focused, not distracted at all by anything'

'You stopped reacting. You didn't react if I interrupted you. You remained calm, focused and repeated what you said until I got it'

'You had no emotional reaction to being interrupted'

'You seemed to be released of judgment about my questions'

'You had no frustration, just focus'

'I felt intrigued by what you were telling me and wanted to know more'

'I didn't feel distracted. It cleared my head of my thoughts about my breakup with Lauren'

For me, I felt the release of distraction of thoughts, I felt the focus, I felt completely present with Jacques and we had an interesting conversation following the exercise about the subject of the paragraph. I felt like my head had been cleared of debris and I'd received a top up of energy. No tension. I felt aware and awake, with a clear view. My breathing even felt opened up, as if I had done a steam Vicks Vaporub with the towel over my head but without the stinging and snotty side effects. I felt ready and inspired to do something else. The exercise was also fun. Like a game that left me feeling as relaxed as if I had had a head massage.

Summary and tips: This is a great exercise for when you are feeling lethargic and slightly tense, or distracted by many thoughts. Do this when you are lacking inspiration and motivation, especially when a friend is visiting.

Day 2: 'writing the wrong' (exercising harmony in disclosure)

It's Sunday. I'm sipping my third coffee, inside the open plan living room overlooking the lake on a windy, grey skies winter day with a log slow burning in the fireplace behind me. I delay beginning the exercise for a few minutes, as there is some tension in my stomach that runs up to my solar plexus and I notice that my shoulders are raised a little. I go to the bathroom, decide to make a cup of coffee. I imagine I'm anxious about transcribing something I have been avoiding for most of my life. Well since I was seven or eight years old.

I take a blank piece of paper and write for five minutes about a specific situation, which represent what I imagine is the most traumatic period of my life. As I write, more examples, more situations that I resent someone for come up. I feel tears forming in my eyes as I remember some images. But at the same time I feel stronger. I realize I am not to blame and that it is not right for me to feel shame. As I continue writing, I come to realize that there are two situations or unresolved resentments from my past that I need to get over before I have a completely clear head, or a clear feeling in my stomach and solar plexus. This clarity of awareness of these two 'dark clouds' that I need to tackle makes me want to take very specific actions to address them both this year.

Honestly, this exercise saddened me by reconnecting with my traumatic experiences, although I feel have delimited issues in my life two very specific main sources of 'trouble'. That awareness, and being able to take actions now, in the present, to address those sources of trouble is already somewhat liberating. It is empowering. The awareness is like as a project manager who keeps track of the project tasks. When presenting to senior management the project manager has a risks and issues slide, which is used as reference tool for tracking mitigating actions that address the risks and issues with different stakeholders. That's exactly what this exercise does, except instead of presenting to senior management, I'm presenting to myself. And because my experience that I wrote about involved another person, I will be using my risks and issues slide on the exercise for day 3…

Summary and tips:
Although upsetting, this exercise is enormously empowering in gaining back control over your life through awareness and being able to do something about the traumatic experiences and sources of shame in life. It helped me to delimit my trauma, trouble and shame to very specific sources, which I can now take steps to address, and get over.

Day 3: 'express myself' (exercising integrity)

Of all the exercises in this book, this one may be the one that saved my life. It helped me to rid myself of false beliefs about myself, beliefs I have held about myself since I was 7 years old. I've been repressing anger and believing lies since then. 30 years. The problem is that I looked up to and believed everything the person I needed to express myself to said, and over time this turned into a core belief about who I am: Useless, nervous, afraid of making a mistake, and as a result, more likely to make a mistake. I have been accident prone as I my anger remains repressed and my fear continues to exist through association. I used alcohol to escape and avoid my fear and my anger. I feel I had to express my resentment in this instance in many ways to save myself from this destructive belief about myself, and it was only when I got it out in the open, in the public domain and in conversation with the person who I had believed all those years ago that I was able to see how truly ridiculous my core belief was.

I chose one evening a day before I was due to travel back to the USA to open the expression session with a question about feeling close to others, and expressing my wish to feel closer to them, without barriers and 'acts'. I explained that I had been acting more stupid than I am around them as a 'cover' and coping mechanism, and that I don't like how my shoulders rise up and tense up around them any time the other person tries to make physical contact with me. I felt a lot of tension in my stomach and an enormous amount of nervous energy running into my chest as I started the conversation. I paused. Just opening the dialogue brought about a sudden emotional rush and I struggled not to let tears overtake me and prevent my clear expression. I then continued riding the energy wave in my body with my surfboard of awareness by expressing some resentments around use of the word 'useless' in specific situations that I can remember from my childhood. After these were expressed I switched to the other person's point of view and felt a lot of empathy and compassion for them, aware of the situation the person was in at the time they called me 'useless' and of the determining influences that had led to them thinking the way they did up to and including that specific point in time. I then felt appreciation and expressed appreciation to them. After about 30 minutes the tension I had felt during the exercise had subsided and the next day the relationship was noticeably more relaxed, open and we were both able to joke together and fool around, something I have not been able to do with this person for a very long time.

Summary and tips:
I feel opening the dialogue by stating the benefit I desired (a closer, more open relationship) for both of us made for a non-confrontational approach that solicited a non-defensive reaction from the subject of my expression. Staying aware of my bodily sensations and not being reactive and caught up to the other person's reactions helped me to stay on task in expressing myself, with the help of pauses. This exercise instantly brought me closer to one of the most important people in my life.

Day 4: 'call it bullshit' (exercising frankness)

I'm at the Goblin café in Summer Hill, Sydney, about to go the centre that organized the 'Happiness and its Causes' world happiness conference, which I worked at last month. The occasion, this Saturday, is an afternoon tea to thank those who helped with the conference. These kinds of social events – just like meetings at work – can be hotspots for egos, masks and second agendas. This exercise is a perfect opportunity for me to clarify my own intention and agenda and try and rid myself of any BS before I enter into conversations at the afternoon tea…

1. What is my intention going into this conversation?
   My intention is to act bold, confident, and improve my chances of confirming a high profile, keynote speaker slot at next year's world happiness conference in Sydney.

2. Am I operating with a second agenda?
   YES. My second agenda is self-promotion (this is second to the agenda of receiving gratitude and enjoying the social event and afternoon tea (of which I am a big fan).

3. What is my real motivation for this conversation?
   Networking, connecting well, creating a situation where the conference organizers want me as a draw card for next year's

conference. Then get asked to speak at the conference. Show off my capabilities as an articulate and charismatic speaker.

After I've answered the above questions and as I'm sitting opposite a vacant chair at my table in the cafe, I have an imaginary conversation with the conference organizer (I put the phone to my mouth so the café staff and publicans don't think I'm insane – it's my ego, there it is). I practice starting my sentences with the words 'I notice' or 'I imagine', then I change the 'I imagine' sentences to begin 'I bullshit'. I give myself permission to be frank and to focus on the sensations in my body that I can actually notice when talking with the conference organizer. Now I've had a good bullshit scrub off, I'm ready for the real conversations, and ready to keep them real. I'm looking forward to reporting back later today on how those conversations go.

*****

I felt a great sense of confidence and no social anxiety as I walked into the centre where the afternoon tea was being held. One of the conference organizers was still making finishing touches to the buffet spread, and I greeted her with a confident resonating voice. And then greeted one of the volunteer organizers, who arrived just after me. As I entered into conversation, I wasn't thinking about or asking myself what was the right thing to say. I spoke more like a child would with an adult's vocabulary, saying what I thought, but also wanting to contribute to and help connect the conversation. The main conference organizer was absent from the tea, but I did get to talk about my book and landed an opportunity to write an article for a magazine. Interestingly, that opportunity came up naturally in conversation, rather than me forcing the agenda. It was more pull than push. And pull had been my intention going into the interaction.

Another side-effect or benefit of the exercise was that I became more aware of the bullshit in other people's words and noticed those who I imagine were saying things to show off knowledge, like peacock feathers, rather than to necessarily contribute something new and authentic to the conversation.

Summary and tips:
Any sentence that begins with 'I' and is an assessment rather than a statement of intention, can be started with either 'I notice' (for thoughts of sensory origin) or 'I imagine' (for thoughts that are not of sensory origin). Noticing whether it's an 'I imagine' or an 'I notice' thought I'm having is a shortcut to identifying a lot of the BS in my head, and prepares me for a real

conversation where I can be clear about my intentions without all the 'I imagine' BS.

Day 5: 'trust myself and trust that I can trust others' (exercising trust)

It's Thursday. I'm sat in a new café in Bondi Junction. The coffee is not as good as what I've been used to at Don Adan and the award winning beans down at the lake house. Hell it's not even as good as home brand Woolworths coffee machine coffee. Yesterday, as I was dropping off my suit pants to be dry cleaned to get the chewing gum off the ass area – an unwanted addition that came from sitting on a bench at Wynyard train station – I spotted a detox business. Given I have been feeling particularly unhealthy in the last week, I was motivated to act spontaneously in response to a billboard advertisement for colon hydrotherapy. I went online on my BlackBerry and found a Groupon, and made an appointment for today at 3:30pm. Now I'm slightly anxious about the prospect of a complete stranger shoving a tube up my ass. I can't think of a better day to exercise trust of myself and others.

Today's exercise is in two parts. Part I is an exercise in trusting myself (pre-colonic). Here are the instructions (taken from *The Happiness Animal*) followed by my observations.

1. Sit or lie down so that you feel comfortable.

   I decided to move from the noisy outdoor location on the street in this café and go back to the house. I am uncomfortable as I need to go to the bathroom. One bathroom break later, I'm now sitting comfortably propped up by large cushions against the bed head.

2. Now, how can you make it even more comfortable? Get a blanket, a pillow... whatever will make you feel relaxed and content.

   I add another blanket and put two pillows behind my head to support my neck. I'm now even warmer and more comfortable.

3. Once you are settled, ask yourself: 'How do I know this is comfortable?' This might appear to be a silly question, and perhaps even confusing. However, it is an important one in increasing your skills of building trust (using your senses, not your mind).

    My breathing has slowed and my muscles feel more relaxed. I'm feeling a little sleepy. My stomach has relaxed and is sticking out a little.

4. Continue to explore what sensation you feel that you recognize as comfort. For example, you might think: 'I do not feel any pain', 'I breathe easily', or 'I feel relaxed'.

    I feel the tingling warmth of a little ASMR (Auto-sensory meridian response) in the back of my head, and my breathing feels unhindered. Warmth. I feel cushioned by the bed.

5. You might be anticipating that this feeling won't last, which is true. We can't control or grasp onto this pleasurable feeling. It's only important that you are in the present moment right now, not drifting into thoughts of the future or the past. Thinking of the future can create anxiety; thinking of the past can create depression.

6. Remain aware of any sounds, the temperature, the light, and your physical sensations. Can you let yourself simply enjoy the moment?

The light in this bedroom is dim, a red glow from the red, Asian lampshade and the cloudy windowpane that opens onto a passageway between this building and next-door. I notice the noise of cars passing outside on a wet road. The temperature is cool, with a little warmth emanating from the heater at the side of the bed.

7. You can practice this exercise for as long as you prefer and as time allows you. Just keep checking in with your level of comfort. What feelings indicate that you are comfortable? With time, you will start to trust your feelings (your senses) again.

I feel myself sinking into the bed, and my toes moving freely back and forth. My breathing feels unhindered. I feel like I'm getting to know what makes me comfortable, and it does feel like I can trust myself a little more. Now I just need to be able to trust someone shoving a tube up my ass.

In The Happiness Animal, Part II of this exercise involves more everyday acts of trust, like asking someone to make me a hot drink of my choice. I'm going a little extreme in my take on Part II, by asking someone to put a tube in my butt, and trusting that they can do it for me without damaging my pipes. Another element to part II is to practice trusting body language, which I will do with a friend. I opted not to do this during colonic hydrotherapy with a stranger.

*****

So it's two days post colonic, and I'm sitting in the sunshine of the Tamarama beach café with the husky by my side again. I'm reflecting now on the body invasion that happened on Thursday. To be honest, as I lay in the bed-cum-toilet, with a stranger explaining that eight gallons of water would be pumped into my lower intestine, and that I needed to hold it in for fifteen seconds before releasing it below the bed, I was fucking scared. The colonic therapist explained I could watch what came out through a three inch, clear plastic tube, in the reflection of a perfectly positioned mirror. My first thought was this is definitely not natural. My next thought was what if I hold it too long and my guts explode and I die of internal bleeding?

****

In the end I didn't need to trust another person inserting the tube in my butt, because that duty fell to me. So I trusted myself and pushed it in a good three inches. Then it required repositioning. Covered with a towel to protect my ever shrinking manhood, I then got my opportunity to trust not one but three women who rotated their entry into the room. I trusted the seemingly new staff member to switch on the flow, but after a couple of minutes and still no sensation of 37.5˚C water flowing between my ass cheeks, my trust began to falter. Enter a more senior staff member who had assumed that I was a seasoned colonicker. Wrong. I had all of a few seconds to trust her before I started to feel the need to poop as liters of warm liquid rushed up into my ass. But as my anxiety subsided, I decided not to pull the tube out of or switch off the water. And to literally ride the flow. Once the eight gallons had been pumped and I'd removed the tube, I felt enormous relief that I had survived, and a renewed pressure in my bowels that resulted in an urge to run to the bathroom. All in all though, I noticed that this hadn't just been an exercise of trust, it was an exercise in facing fear and the unknown, and for that reason I felt double the mild euphoria as I walked home. I also felt lighter, more energetic and more alive. Two days later, I'm still feeling the benefits. But one colonic experience in my lifetime is enough. That said, I still feel like I didn't really fully exercise part II of the trusting others exercise. But moments after leaving the café, I needed to use the bathroom. Rather than take the husky into the bathroom with me I asked a trustworthy man in a group of four others, who was holding a camera if he could hold my rucksack, which was attached to the leash and the husky dog, and held my wallet, my new phone and my laptop. Valuable possessions and a great opportunity for trusting a stranger. It worked. Even as I went to the bathroom I felt lighter and refreshed, and this before I relieved myself and spent a penny. I then got the back wave of energy and smiles as I returned to retrieve the husky, backpack, and belongings. In the minute I'd been gone, it seemed the man had already formed a bond with the husky, and looked even a little reluctant to say goodbye, although when he did, he did so with a smile. Inadvertently it seemed that I'd helped him exercise his happiness muscle with protection, kindness and compassion.

Summary and tips: Part II can involve planning but be open to spontaneous opportunities to exercise trust. These trusting exercises produce feelings of lightness of body and mind, relaxation, general well being and ease.

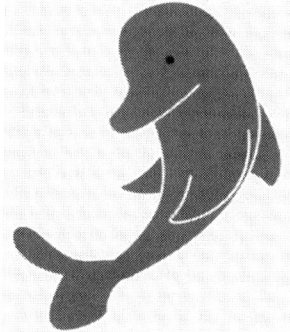

Chapter 2

Five days kind

The spirit in which a present is given is more important than the present itself

Seneca

There is no choice between being kind to others and being kind to ourselves. It is the same thing

Piero Ferrucci

Before I began work on *The Happiness Animal* my kindness muscle was in atrophy. Why would I do something for someone else when I could do something for myself? I put my self-interests first. I was selfish. Doing something for someone else almost always seemed counter-intuitive to doing something for myself. Little did I know that the most I could do to help myself was to help or to be kind to others. Once I understood that being kind was in my interest, I became instantly attracted to using the daily opportunities for kindness that would spring up to help myself feel useful, connected to others, and happier! *Yes mum, I will drive granny to the supermarket to get her shopping. Here let me help you carry that, I'm walking this way too. Here, you look like you could use a tissue. I'll cook dinner for you and dad tonight. You look like you are in a rush and you only have a couple of items to pay for so you go before me in the queue.* Some days I forget the simple truth that being kind makes me happy. I want some daily exercise to stay fit and keep my kindness connection healthy. With that, I'm going to start my five days of kindness. Oh, and here's a final reminder that if you want to try the exercises I'm doing yourself, they can all be found in the back of this book in the appendix section.

Day 6: '4 smiles, 4 hugs and a cup of tea' (exercising warmth)

Time for some honesty first: I found myself doing this exercise across three days rather than one. In practice there are three exercises and the benefits of each are enough to keep happiness muscles exercised enough for one day, though I imagine doing all three in one day would be a day of happiness and not much else. The cup of tea part came first. I was at a train station in England on my way to book my trip from Penzance to London when I spotted a girl in tears outside of the ticket office. I walked up to her and asked, 'hey what's the matter?' She sobbed and said that she'd missed her train back to London, that she was so stupid and that she was leaving her friend behind and wouldn't be able to get back here again for a long time, and that she couldn't afford another ticket back to London. It was also raining heavily outside the station and her clothing and hair were both half drenched. I said, 'sometimes shit happens and it feels like it's the end of the world but really this will pass and this really isn't the end of the world even though it feels like it is. Do you want a hug?' I gave her a hug and she half laughed. Then I said, come on let's get you a cup of tea. It'll make you feel better. We walked into the café inside the station, and I asked her what kind of tea she'd like and ordered it and paid. Then we went back out onto the platform where she could wait for the next train. By now her tears were dried and she looked at me, smiled and said thank you. I said good luck and smiled back. After I walked out of the station I would never see her again. But I had felt a lot of warmth, gratitude and it made me feel connected for a long time. In fact the good feelings from this one brief interaction stuck around for several months. It more than made my day to do a simple act of warmth and connect with another human being.

For the hugs and smiles, these are a lot easier to incorporate into every day. In fact I believe every day would be a lot better if we did. I also feel like I get double the benefit if I make a note of each smile and hug in an email to myself on my phone. That way I get reminders of what went well each day, and I get to feel a little more appreciation, gratitude and connectedness to my day and to others even after the act itself. For this exercise though, I decided to do all my hugs in one go. There were three people working at the café I've been visiting in Bowral in the last week, so I approached one of the staff and said 'I've got an unusual request. I'm writing a book about happiness and doing exercises each day and writing about how each exercise makes me feel. Today's part of the exercise is to give four people a hug'. I got the reply, 'we can do that'.
So two of the cafe staff came out from behind the counter, the first with reaching open arms and an Adidas T-shirt and I responded with an immediate embrace. The next one was waiting for her turn, and after the second hug I turned around to see where the third girl was and she was walking towards me with urgency as if she didn't want to risk missing out on her hug. Then I said, 'I like this café'. We were all beaming smiles and I walked out to go catch my train feeling connected and somewhat elated from the concentrated dose of human warmth. A triple shot of happiness juice. For the fourth hug of the day I knew I'd be meeting a new person that evening, someone whose house and hound I'd be looking after for the next two weeks so it was a safe bet that I'd be able to hug her upon meeting, which I did. That way I got another shot towards the end of the day to keep me pepped up.

Now here's my smile log for the day:
Smile 1: Mother at a table with two other mothers of infants. 11:30 am.

Smile 2: Retired man in the café. 12:28 pm.
The more I'm smiling the more confident I'm feeling looking at strangers. I feel more relaxed after this second smile.

Smile 3: Old lady in the café sat at a table on her own. 12:50 pm.
This prompted a long lasting smile, which I could see in my peripheral vision after I had turned away and I felt a sense of calm. After this smile I'm also getting a strong appreciation of the people I am smiling at as unique individuals and I'm starting to see a unique story behind each pair of smiling eyes. Each smile feels like a brief yet almost intimate connection with a stranger, a nonverbal communication that almost says 'I know you and I see you'. I'm surprised at the depth of response I'm feeling from something this simple.

Smile 4: Smiled at the male waiter in the café when he was asking me whether two glasses and a half-full bottle of water were mine. 1.10 pm.
I felt yet even more relaxed in the café after this smile. Time to leave the café and go enjoy some sunshine.

Summary and tips:
This is a good exercise for when you are feeling lonely, cold, or isolated. This warms up your daily routine and reconnects you to the world of other people.

Day 7: 'hear me now' (exercising respect)

Before I did this exercise I was waiting for a train in the Southern Highlands of Australia. A short, fifty-something, long haired man (think Game of Thrones villager crossed with a Hobbit) with a few days of grime on skin, and a few days of grease in hair, dirty T-shirt and darkened jeans, came up to me as I leant against the top the backrest of a bench facing the sun, while I snacked on some raw broccoli. My train wasn't coming for another twenty minutes. My instinct was to avoid conversation with him but then I remembered I wanted to do this listening exercise. So I pflunged my thoughts lever to off, took some deep breaths and focused all my attention on the man, looking him square in the eyes. Let's call him Throdo. Throdo started muttering something about a pale twenty-something year old man with a plastic leg brace on the platform opposite, about twenty meters away, who was using sign language to ask the Throdo if he had a 'stick' (Aussie code for joint). The pale man got up and then keeled over like he was about to vomit on his grocery bags on the platform.

'He's on something. He could get arrested asking for drugs on a train platform. I've never seen him before. If he comes over here, will you give him the bullet?' asked Throdo.

'What do you mean? Give him the bullet?' I asked closing my bag of broccoli to focus on the conversation.

'You know, tell him to get lost. I lived on the street for twenty-five years so you know I know how to handle myself. If he tries anything with me....well....see that branch on that tree?'

'Oh you mean that big branch, is that right?' I asked.

'Yep, I can carry one of those under each arm'.

'How old you are you?' asked Throdo.

Thirty-seven,' I replied.

'See you're bigger. We are men. He's just a pale kid. A user. If he comes over here (as Throdo spoke, the pale man appeared to be struggling to get into the lift on the other side of the platform) and gives us any shit, I'm going to ask him, is your name candlestick?'

'Candlestick?' I asked.

'Yep one blow and he's out,' he chuckled.

'Did you like that one?' Throdo asked. 'You can take that back to England with you'.

'I will remember that one, thanks'.

'Yep, I should go to England and do some standup comedy over there. Here's another one for you...'

'Why doesn't anyone in Iraq have a television? Because of the Teleban. Ha-ha'.

'Did you like that one?' He repeated. You can take that back to England with you'.

'Ha-ha, Yes I'll remember that one. Teleban. Thanks'.

Shortly after, the man boarded the train and disappeared forever. But for ten minutes I really listened to his tales and attempts at humor.

That night, I continued my listening exercise with the owner of the house and hound I was looking after for the next 2 weeks. She decided to take me out for dinner as a thank you on my first night before she left the next day. Over dinner I practiced paraphrasing back with phrases like 'so you were in a cab on the harbor bridge on the way back from your the oncologist appointment, and you had just told your boss you'd just been diagnosed with cancer, and while you were in the cab, he told you that you were fired. Is that right?'

My default is to simply listen, nod, and interject with 'wow' and nods, and 'yes' and 'no', but I felt much more connected to the speaker and the conversation when I asked questions to confirm my understanding and paraphrased back. Simply by asking 'is that right?' at the end of my sentences, I felt more awake, more present, and more connected to the conversation. I'm going to try to incorporate some more paraphrasing and ending my sentences with 'is that right?' as a result of this exercise.

Summary and tips:
One of the easiest ways to connect with a conversation partner (and to engage the muscle for active listening) is by asking simple questions and by paraphrasing back what they say to confirm and demonstrate understanding. This exercise woke me up, connected me, energized me and grounded me.

Day 8: 'I appreciate you' (exercising recognition and appreciation)

Just thinking about doing this exercise with a stranger fills me with an ASMR-like rush of warmth, similar to self-administering a small dose of morphine, but without the side effects. You know that feeling you got when you were a child in bed with your head on the pillow and your mother brushed your hair back behind your ear with her hand, or when your grandfather was reading you a story.

Per exercise instructions, I identify an individual. It's Monday lunchtime and I'm at the Don Adan café where I wrote much of my first book, *The Happiness Animal*. I'm looking at the new barista in the café. Next, I list 3 body movements I notice in the individual:
1) I notice the way he casually has his hand in one pocket as he moves around in the kitchen.

2) I notice his relaxed posture, with his knee resting against side of the kitchen, and his hands resting on his thighs when he's moving around and then with one hand in the pocket.

3) I notice his subtle, understated smile and his neck leaning forward.

Next, I list one of his body movements or positions I also notice as similar in myself: the one hand in the pocket.

Then I list a description of the barista that I appreciate him for: I appreciate his calm tone with slight smile when he is talking. I make eye contact with him, smile and tell him what I appreciate him for. It was definitely awkward, but my comment was gratefully received and the response was 'I'm glad you appreciate it'. I felt connected and not in a flirtatious way. Just at ease, relaxed. And it was a great icebreaker. After a comment of appreciation it seemed to open the floor for any dialogue except small talk.

Summary and tips:
Looking for what I appreciate in others is a sure and fast way to raise my spirits. It's the antidote to demoralizing selfishness and a feeling of isolation. Vocalizing the appreciation can be an uncomfortable yet extremely connecting and rewarding experience. The perfect ice breaker.

Day 9: 'A tissue!' (exercising kindness with the ABC of gratitude)

The ABC of gratitude is the Altruism, Benefits and Consideration of Gratitude. The idea of this exercise is, when in a public place, to be on the lookout for anyone whom you anticipate would benefit from you giving him or her a tissue for any reason. It could be tears, a runny nose, a spillage-on-self situation, or otherwise. I was once the recipient of a stranger's tissue on a train in Sydney when I was suffering from a runny nose. I was struck by how much of an impact the simple gift and interaction from a stranger – and my resultant gratitude – had on my sense of wellbeing. Even to the point of feeling warmth, increased relaxation and general ease of being. I also noticed how natural and real the smile on the giving stranger's face was immediately following this simple interaction. So I decided to repeat the exercise, but this time with my role as the giving stranger. The first time I tried this exercise was in a suburb of Melbourne at the Coles supermarket. I saw a woman leaving the store through the automatic doors, and as she walked off I asked her, 'would you like a tissue?' It felt extremely forced and unnatural, and I was uncomfortable to the point of feeling like I was doing something illegal. After a concerned look followed by a 'no, thank you,' I walked into the supermarket and had a chuckle to myself as I realized that any potential tissue recipient would have to have a clearly identifiable, immediate need for assistance, otherwise I would freak them out.

Take two and I'm on a train from Melbourne to Sydney. As I regularly do on train journeys, I indulged in a little conversation with my neighboring passengers. During the initial stages of the conversation I mentioned that the reason why I kept scouring the carriage with a hawk eye, was that I was trying out an exercise for my book where I'd hopefully increase my sense of wellbeing by giving someone in need, a tissue. I was disappointed when I spotted a napkin on my neighbor's table and realized she wouldn't need a tissue to wipe her face after eating her food from the buffet car. The two women suggested with a giggle that their friend, who was sat at the back of the carriage with her mother could do with a tissue. Apparently she was 'edgy' having not been allowed to have a cigarette for the last four hours, and was a likely candidate for bursting into tears at any point during the journey. As I made my way to the toilet I passed the friend they'd been talking about. The two women had got up from their seats and walked down to said friend. One of the women asked the friend if she needed a tissue and then told her and her mother the story of my tissue antics on train. Then, the mother of the friend said she might need a tissue when she sees her son at his graduation tomorrow. So I asked her, 'would you like a tissue?' The conversation and the tissue were more a source of amusement than a genuine exercise of altruism, benefits and consideration in this instance. That said, this exercise did still help me and others to connect better with each other and made for a not-insignificantly-happier journey for at least five of us.

Following this interaction a passenger boarded the train in Albury and sat in the vacant seat next to me. This passenger was genuinely sniffing and I got another chance to ask if they wanted a tissue. But again the answer was no. But then, twenty minutes later came my chance to fulfill the exercise in line with my original intention. The quieter of the two women neighboring me spilt milk on her black pants and so there was a real and immediate need for assistance. In this instance I offered the whole pack of tissues, which was greeted by laughter, 'thank you' and I felt a real sense of warmth in my upper gut into my chest. Again came the sense of relaxation that I call 'ease of being' that I'd experienced as a recipient of a tissue during my own sniffy moment. What I ultimately experienced as the giver was a feeling of being *useful* to others. And it's this being useful to others, which is happiness gold.

In reality it can be a lot harder than I had expected to find someone in a public place who actually needs a tissue. So I'd recommend substituting the tissue with a more general approach. Start with the intention of looking for an individual in a public place whose need can be anticipated, and then provide them with a benefit that considers that need. The benefit, I imagine, needs to be something more significant than moving out the way on the train while another passenger carries foods past, and more significant than holding the door open for someone. The benefit needs to be something as specific as the tissue (but not necessarily the tissue) for it to be well considered enough to constitute acting out of an intention of altruism, and not mere politeness or good will. What also seemed to help, if you decide to stick with the tissue giving, is to first communicate to others that you have an available benefit. By telling the neighboring passengers about my exercise and the benefits I could offer them, when the need for the benefit arose they anticipated that I could help them. They were primed, prepared and ready to accept my help. And they were grateful once they had received my benefit. Of course this strategy can also be adopted as much in the workplace as it can in the train carriage.

Summary and tips:
You don't need a tissue to exercise the ABC of Gratitude. Notice a need and consider what would be a benefit. And if possible, communicate what you are able to help with before the need arises. This is an excellent exercise for connecting well with strangers and offers reprieve from feelings of homesickness, isolation or loneliness while travelling.

Day 10: 'Musical chairs' (exercising empathy)

It's Saturday morning the sun is shining on the lake – a nice day for a white wedding. I appreciate nature, the sunshine, the clean air. Although deep down there are some lingering stinky prawns of resentment that I need to purge myself of before I fully appreciate each new day. It's like knowing that there is bulldog clip inside my stomach, squeezing a small part of my gut. I'd like to take it off before I go roam the land in the sunshine. Before I feel I can fully enjoy the outside, go clear out rotten apples from under the trees or walk the dog down the trail to the river, I'd like to rid myself of the resentment in me. The only problem is that I am thousands of miles away from the object of my resentment. I'm not even in the same hemisphere. Ideally, I'd express myself with the exercise that came on day three, in person and face-to-face, to get complete with the past and get over it. But when face-to-face resentment is not possible, empathy is. So that's exactly what I'm going to exercise today. I'm going to empathize with the person I resent. And then I'm going to exercise compassion, and even if I can't get rid of that bulldog clip completely, I will at least loosen its grip on my gut.

I start by arranging two chairs facing each other. I sit in one chair imagining the other person is sat in the chair opposite. I have some notes from my resentment exercise that I use to guide me. I start talking to the empty chair. I stop feeling silly after the first couple of sentences and it feels remarkably similar to having a real conversation with someone, with the same uncomfortableness of a real life, hard conversation. I tell the imaginary him that I want to talk to him as a favor to me so I can get over some things, and so I can stop avoiding him, bring us closer. I can imagine that he didn't know what he was doing when he said the things he said and was a lot younger and that in his position I would have said the same, so while I forgive him and don't blame him for acting the way he did, I still want to resent him for the specific things he said, to get it out of my system. I share some specific resentments. Very specific. What time of day it was where it was, even the seat I was sat in, and down to the specific word that I resent him for using: 'useless'. I tell him that I believed and trusted what he said to me and looked up to him as a role model for strength, power and knowledge. As I vocalize some more resentments I start crying, and feel immense sadness as I feel the tears coming. More tears come when I say I want to get complete with this so we can be closer, not distant. At the moments where I feel he would probably jump in and say something I switch seats and imagine I'm him and what he would say back to me, looking at me in the seat I was sat in. I feel his shock, I feel his not knowing what to say, feel how exposed he must feel, that he can't genuinely remember the things I resent him for. I get up and respond back as myself. I tell him I love him too and I want to put this behind us. 'Thank you for listening to me,' I say. I get up and give him a hug. I feel his confusion and helplessness. I feel sorry for him and want to help him. I feel my relationship got closer to him through this exercise even though this was just a virtual, imaginary conversation. I feel more confident about having this tough conversation with him face to face.

Whilst the tears have taken their toll on me and left me a little drained, I do feel buoyed and relieved that my relationship with the other person is more alive. It's a relief that I no longer have to hide my feelings. And more of a relief that I don't have to hide, even if it is scary surfing that big emotional wave all the way to the shore. It is worth noting that by around 3pm in the afternoon, all my sadness had left me and I felt elated for the rest of the day, laughing out loud at nature, smiling and chuckling with the dog. When I saw the many stars and Venus and Jupiter in the sky that night, I felt joy at experiencing the experience of witnessing some of the infinity that is the universe.

There are some additional steps in the exercise still using the two chairs, but now, for exercising compassion: I choose to use the same person to exercise compassion with and also choose my grandmother as well, who is currently suffering from severe arthritis and memory problems. When empathizing with the suffering of both people, one of the emotions I felt consistently was a longing for connection from both people. When I imagined I was either person, I felt like I was alone and I wanted a hug. I wanted someone to talk to and to ask for help. Someone to help me work it all out. When I reached the step of wanting their suffering to end, and then imagined doing something to ease their suffering, I felt a sense of strength, almost as if I could feel strength in the muscles, especially in my arms. I felt conviction and I felt useful, like my purpose was to help them both. That sense of belonging, connection and usefulness, is incredibly life affirming and courage building. I found this compassion exercise useful for practicing things I can say to improve my relationships and help the people I exercised compassion with to connect better with their own existence, and to help relieve their suffering. The exercise got me to vocalizing very specific sentences, which I'd like to use in real, face to face conversation.

The final step of this exercise is to practice doing something small every day to help end the suffering of others, by imagining what the other person would want someone else or me to do to help. So for today's small act to help end the suffering of others I choose to research arthritis and brain supplements and to get something sent to my grandmother as soon as possible. I get a warm feeling. I imagine that's familial love.

Summary and tips
Exercise can be painful, unpleasant and uncomfortable while I'm doing it, but it is afterwards that I begin to feel that sense of strength and satisfaction with my health, and the same goes for this exercise.

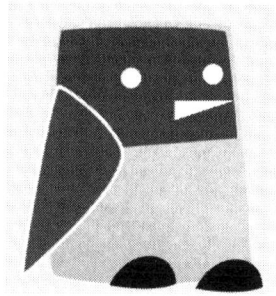

Chapter 3

Five days tolerant

Nothing need arouse one's irritation so long as one doesn't make it bigger than it is by getting irritated

Seneca

Mood goes up mostly with increased tolerance in the nation

Martin Seligman

To understand all is to forgive all

F. Lacordaire

The happiest states of the US are the most tolerant

Livescience

Tolerance is a virtue because it takes human beings very seriously, recognizing that without the freedom to err people can never acquire the freedom to discover truths

Frank Furedi

Bang! The light bulb above my desk exploded showering me with glass. My hi-fi silenced, cutting off Lana Del Rey mid *Diet Mountain Dew*. It was 2012. I was living in a share house in Sydney. I walked out of my room and saw through my housemate Mishka's open room door, him kneeling on the floor, unplugging his fan heater. 'I'll go and switch the power back on,' I said.

'Thanks man,' said Mishka, picking up his longneck of Coopers Red beer from the floor and taking a swig.

I walked down to the fuse box by the kitchen door, and sure enough, the switch had been tripped. I went back upstairs and looked at the calendar on my bedroom door. It was the fifteenth of October. I knew the electricity meter would be read on the seventeenth and the bill would soon follow. My breath quickened. I felt my lungs closing, reducing in size, losing capacity. My two body balloons were trapped in a vice, and no matter how long I tried to make my breaths, I couldn't prise the vice apart. I couldn't work out how much electricity my three housemates and I had used since the last, mammoth bill but when I had called the electricity company midway through the quarter, they had told me that the total usage was already double what it had been for the first bill of the year.

I wish Belle hadn't asked me to look after the electricity for the house, they'll blame me, I thought. My eyebrows tightened and thickened. I imagined my housemates' reactions to the bill. I visualized their faces of few words and few facial movements above rigid bodies that would march down the wooden floors from the kitchen to their rooms, closing their doors with the calculated force that would mask a fully expressed slam. These thoughts slipped my lungs further into the vice, up to my collar bone. *What if Belle refuses to pay me?* I thought. *I have two thousand dollars coming off my credit card in November, and I don't have any money left..., I really don't know what I am going to do.* Since I had looked at the calendar, I had forgotten about my plans for going kayaking that day, forgotten about the coffee machines I had sold and needed to take to the post office. My thoughts began to grasp for potential ways to explain the high bill to help me justify it to my housemates. *I'll never be able to prove it was their heaters that caused it, and they will blame me because I'm the only one at home in the daytime. I don't know how to stop the next bill from being high either, I can't do this,* I thought.

I looked at my to do list, and felt the panic of being stuck in a pit with a truck overhead burying me with cement. 'The customer is still waiting for me to post the coffee machine. Oh shit,' I said. I started boxing up a coffee machine when I felt a pulse of pain behind my ear above the back my jaw. Pain spasmed again and raced, twinging to the back of my head. I winced. I wondered if I could feel pressure behind my eyeballs. I pushed my fingers into my face below my eye socket, closed my eyes, and then palmed my eyeballs, waiting for any deeper pain to emerge. 'Has my headache stopped now?' I asked. 'I can't feel it now can I? Wait, there it is again. Damn it, do I have any painkillers?'

*****

A week later, my headaches had subsided, as had my questioning of whether or not I was getting abnormal sensations of pressure behind my eyeballs. On my phone I could see I had received an email from Dodo with the latest electricity bill attached but I decided to wait until after lunch to look at it. I opened the attachment, and saw the figure was even higher than the previous bill, which had taken everyone by surprise: this time it was one thousand, one hundred and twenty dollars of doom.
'Shit, I need to get the money off Belle and Mishka before that gets taken off my credit card. I need to get the message out now,' I said. Ko walked downstairs, confirmed that no one else was in the house and thumb-typed a group text message on the keyboard of my BlackBerry with the amount and my bank details. Then I ran out of the house to the bus stop and boarded the first bus to the city. My phone vibrated against the bus seat. As I opened the text from Belle I felt an ice rod pierce my solar plexus. Before I had read a word, I could feel my heart palpitating in my temples. My beats per minute were rising, pumping the pace of my blood-flow. I looked at the text. Key words and phrases flashed at me from a blur of screen: *can't understand why it's so high*; *can't afford it; we need to switch provider*; *other provider was cheaper*; *it's because we are on peak now*. I knew that the last of these statements was false. I felt like I'd had a triple latte and it pumped fresh muscle into my mind. Here was my chance to prove I was right. I started typing on the phone at a rate that would meet minimum words per minute requirements for a typist on a full keyboard. Anger, adrenalin, this was flight or fight. I punched these words back at Belle: *We've always been on a single tariff rate. We still have the same old meter we've always had.* Belle replied within a minute: *Well I used to work at Ausgrid and I phoned them up. They said we were on peak so you can see why I'd think that.*
My forehead tightened around the edges and pushed up a mound above my nose. My fingers snapped into reply: *The first bill we got from Dodo was cheaper than the old provider*. Then I napalm texted a triple bombardment to finish the job: *I spent several days researching the rates and Dodo is the cheapest. The reason for the high bill is we've been using more electricity.*

There can't be any doubt that it's because of the fan heater in Mishka's room.

I got back from the city at around 9pm. I was about to plate up my dinner when Mishka arrived and lent his bicycle against the wall outside the kitchen. Mishka took off his helmet to reveal the redness of his forehead and hair dampened down with sweat. He walked into the kitchen where I, body frozen, greeted him with a bug eyed half-grin that said 'well...'

'Just so I understand, or well help me to understand, I'm just getting really frustrated by this whole electricity thing. Can we just break the contract and switch to another provider? We never had any of this shit with the previous provider,' said Mishka

I received a full-face injection of red-heat-righteousness; pressure came in a tsunami behind my lips that could hold it for only seconds before bursting.

'You're frustrated by the electricity? I have the triple fucking frustration of dealing with all this bullshit and coordinating with everyone else in the house. It's bloody ridiculous, if you want to switch provider, there is a fee to break the contract, but if you want to switch provider, go ahead, just the new contract will need to be in your name,' I said, my voice uncharacteristically raised. I looked at my hands trying to gauge whether or not Mishka would notice them trembling. Mishka walked upstairs to his room, closing the door behind him, leaving me shaking in the kitchen, my heart pounding. I had lost control of my body.

****

I have done more than enough reactive napalm-texting (Nobel Prize winning psychologist Daniel Kahneman calls this system one, automatic thinking, or thinking fast at its worst). I'm equally as guilty of wanting to find a scapegoat for a problem that only really existed in my head. And for being unreasonable and angry, rather than aware, calm and collected when faced with people's questions about a high bill. After my accident, PTSD and OCD symptoms amplified my reactive behavior. Fortunately a clinical psychologist named Lauren McNamara asked me specific questions, which helped me understand that my way of thinking was counterproductive to my existence, and that the hell full of never ending problems that I created in my head was entirely imagined by me. Problems only existed as long as I called them problems. They didn't need to be problems and I didn't need to react to them in the way I was. I could survive and be able to live with the worst-case scenario of no one paying me their electricity share. I could survive missing a credit card bill repayment. And I could do things that were possible to prevent that from happening, rather than going into free-fall panic when I received a bill, or even when I just knew that a bill was on its way.

Perhaps tolerance is the one muscle I have improved the health of the most, given I suffered from anxiety, depression, PTSD and OCD and overcame them all through curious exploration of my thinking habits with the help of a psychologist. I am now much more tolerant than I was even before I had the accident, and almost as curious as I was when I was a child. But I don't want to become complacent. I'd love to keep my tolerance connection open and well exercised. It helps in many areas of my life from keeping my demoralizing ego in check (making intolerant judgments in response to difference, or to people saying unexpected things) to not freaking out or becoming panicky or anxious when something doesn't go according to plan or how I had intended it to. With renewed enthusiasm, I'm ready to kick off my five days of exercising tolerance…

Day 11: 'Life through a lens. From telephoto to wide angle' (exercising tolerance with fear)

It's Saturday, it's sunny, and the lake is beautifully still. Birdsong and crickets. I've been enjoying the morning, sipping coffee in the sunshine and applying for jobs in New York, whilst surrounded by tranquility. But nestled in my guts is a fear that wakes from time to time like a baby that stirs in the upstairs bedroom. Then you know it wants feeding. My fear wants to be fed. I'm worried my body suffered from the amount of drinking I did in my not-too-distant past. I'm worried alcohol has taken its toll on my body. I'm worried about my liver. My physical health does seem to be fine but anytime I get the slightest pain in my abdomen or if I imagine I can see a hint of yellow in my eye, I freak out and wonder if my past will come back to get my body. So it's perfect timing for me to exercise tolerance of my fear.

I take a blank sheet of paper and write *fear of liver problems/cirrhosis* in the middle. I follow the exercise instructions and, with a pencil draw circles one at a time around my fear. I notice how the circles are forced to get larger each time and squeeze the space out of the paper until they become all consuming. I realize this is what has been happening in my mind. The more attention I give the fear, the more I feed it, the more it dominates my being, my sheet of paper. I continue to follow the instructions and erase the circles one by one until I am left with only the words of my fear. Using the free space that was previously taken up by my unnecessary circles I write down the name of my girlfriend. I write down that I would enjoy making love, walking, talking and cooking with her. And that I'd like help coach her for auditions. I write down that I can do these things activities with her in July, when I return to New York from Australia. I write down my grandparents and that I'd like to cook for them and stock their cupboards with some health foods that may help with their arthritis, in the summer. I look back at my fear in the middle of the piece of paper and realize that all the circles I drew around it were unnecessary, and they were not leaving space for the good things in my life. I laugh at myself. I feel somewhat relieved, lighter like some of the weight has been taken from my stomach, and I feel buoyed by wanting to do what I want to do for my girlfriend and my grandparents.

I reality test my fear. The worst that can happen is I have cirrhosis. I estimate there is a 3/10 likelihood I have it, but writing this down I imagine it is closer to 2/10. I can reduce the likelihood of getting it by eating healthily, not drinking alcohol and avoiding anything with toxins in it. And yes, it's even possible that I can survive cirrhosis if the worst did happen.

Summary and tips: This exercise was very useful at getting me out of my head and showing me the wonderful world all around. It reduced the amount of attention I gave to my fear and helped me focus on what I can do to help others, which I know will make me happier.

Day 12: 'Breath easy' (exercising tolerance of pain)

It's Monday morning. I'm a little anxious about finding a place to live, which I am currently doing through house-sitting. My potential next house-owner has asked me for references and police checks, which I am trying to figure out how to obtain. This request was unexpected and has disrupted my plans for today. Right around the same time, I also start feeling a little pain behind my eyeballs, discomfort in the back of my head, and in my cheeks, as well as tightness in the front of my head and my stomach. While the pain is far from severe, it is an opportunity to test out this exercise.

I'm finding it difficult to think about anything other than how much tension I'm feeling. The pre-exercise task is to complete the following sentence: If I didn't feel pain, what feeling would I be left with right now? Here's my answer: A relaxed all over body sensation, lightness in my body, in my cheeks and soothing calm. I then complete the breathing exercise (see page 165), but to be honest with you, I stopped feeling discomfort by the time I'd completed step four. I will come back to this exercise when I feel more intense pain.

Summary and tips:
For light pain, tension and discomfort, spending a couple of minutes getting to step four (see page 165) of this exercise was enough. Perhaps increasing the steps is akin to increasing the dose of the painkiller.

Day 13: 'All in the same boat' (exercising tolerance of others)

Before I start this exercise, I am in a café in Bowral, a small town in the Southern Highlands about two hours drive south of Sydney, Australia. A girl walks past the long table where I am currently sitting writing this and opens the café door, which is next to me. This is on a winter's day with an outside temperature around 45'F (7'C). The girl then walks back to her table where she is ostensibly sitting with her family members. I notice that everyone in her group (including the girl) is wearing a heavy winter coat. My first reaction to her opening the door is disdain and wanting to shut the door immediately. Cut to the next day. Another café. This time I'm sitting outside in the winter sun. I have my exercise steps at the ready. I start scouting the café for a target person. I notice a middle aged man wearing Oakley sunglasses, hands in his pocket, silent, motionless and emotionless, sat opposite a woman I assume to be his wife. I look at him. I notice my reaction. It is a frown. Now his arms are crossed. I resent him for his sunglasses, his crossed arms, his posture, his lack of animation and his silence with his wife. I notice the physical sensations in my body. They are: tension in my forehead, stomach, and tightness in my chest. I pay attention to those sensations for thirty seconds and they diminish quickly.

I then repeat to myself:
      a. 'Just like me, this person is seeking happiness in his/her life.'

    b. 'Just like me, this person is trying to avoid suffering in his/her life.'

    c. 'Just like me, this person has known sadness, loneliness and despair.'

    d. 'Just like me, this person is seeking to fill his/her needs.'

    e. 'Just like me, this person is learning about life.'

Wow! As I'm repeating these phrases to myself, I feel a rush of warmth and love for this man, who I resented for his sunglasses and crossed arms only moments before. I look back at him. I notice that he is now talking to his wife. And even a little smile emerges on his face. He takes money out of his wallet to pay for drinks and hands it to his wife. I realize that I take money out and hand it to my girlfriend in the same way. I notice that I look around the café in the same way he does. I recognize the similarities between his and my own body movements. And I notice that his jeans are a bit droopy and need pulling up around the waist, just like mine do sometimes. I notice that my own sensations of tension that I felt when I first laid eyes upon this man have changed. I am no longer tense but freed from judgment. I feel relaxed and a little joy. I feel happier.

Summary and tips:
Judging others by appearance almost always (if not always) demoralizes me. Noticing my reaction of judgment or disdain is a great trigger to remember the antidote: Simply by repeating the above phrases I neutralized animosity and demoralizing tension in my body.

Day 14: 'A plant, a jug, five mugs and a teaspoon' (exercising patience)

It's Sunday, the farm I'm staying at has a bushfire awareness event with a bouncy castle, food and drinks about fifty yards back from the lake house where I am sat writing this. I'm curious to explore the event, not wanting to miss the opportunity for some human contact (and the chance to have some free food). Since I've been here in the lake house, house sitting for 3 weeks now, most of my time has been solitary, my main contact limited to looking after the Chihuahua and nineteen year old cat. As you can imagine, after this drought of human contact I'm almost impatient to go say hello to those people here, even if it is only in passing as I take the recycling to the sheds or the food scraps to the pigs. I am impatient, which made sitting down to write this all the less appealing, especially after three coffees. But as I do write I can feel myself already becoming a little less impatient. The energy around the front of my forehead, the tension in my ribs and leg muscles is relaxing a little, and is curbing my instinct to bound out of the house.

Before I began work on The Happiness Animal, I was even more impatient than I am now. I also had a notoriously short attention span and regularly became distracted by emails, messages, noises inside or outside, or by random ideas to do something else that flashed through my chain of thoughts and thinking links like fireworks saying 'hey dude! Come watch us!' So with this morning's reminder of my tendency for impatience in mind, I can think of no better opportunity than now to exercise some patience. I follow my own instructions and get a jug, five mugs and a teaspoon and decide to use the small vegetable and herb garden at the back of the property as the setting for my exercise. First, I fill five mugs to the brim with water from the tap in the back kitchen next to the espresso machine, although not before I am momentarily distracted by gunshots from across the lake and see kangaroos bouncing up the hill, jumping for their lives to escape whoever it is who is trying to kill them. Back to filling the five mugs... As I carry the mugs one by one to the plants, feelings similar to those I'd experienced during the connecting with words exercise (for sincerity) come to me. I feel focused on right now; my senses are sharpened. I notice each breath that I take, and breathe deeply and easily so as not to spill the water. I imagine I enjoy the activity more because of the novelty of it not having a purpose. Sure it's watering the plants but I don't need to water the plants (they are getting enough rain) and I could just do it with a hose or with a watering can. By the time I pick up the fifth mug, I feel an ASMR-type warmth and relaxation flood my temples. I can compare it to the feeling I got when was able to self-administer morphine (although without the side effects and to a much lesser degree).

I have already felt the positive effects from filling and careful and patiently moving the mugs, so when it comes to emptying them with a teaspoon, I question (the thought runs through my head) whether I can just tip the mugs out or leave them full. A dart of impatience runs through my temples. But by the time I start tea spooning out the third mug, I become more present and focused again as the thoughts that this is a waste of time clear from my head. I also find that simply looking into the water, whether in the teaspoon or especially in the mug, to be incredibly soothing. Perhaps that's why we find peace staring out at the horizon across the ocean or sitting on the shore of a river. I notice if I speed up the spooning to the plant or spill any, I don't enjoy what I am doing as much. If I look at the brimming spoon, it calms me again. My senses become fine tuned so that I can notice the feeling of water rushing around the spoon when I put it in the mug, and the difference in weight in the spoon with the water in it compared to when it is empty. It is only on the fifth mug that I become aware of the clink of the spoon on the mug and that I like the sound of it. I also start looking at the plant as if it am appreciating me spoon-feeding it, and somehow the spoon feels more alive, almost connected to me.

In the house there is a large water filtration dispenser with a removable reservoir inside the top of the unit. I realize that I have been filling it with a small jug rather than taking it to the sink and filling it directly from the tap, because I like doing it the slow way. I like filling the jug, then the reservoir, rather than just filling the reservoir. I enjoyed this exercise a lot more than I imagined I would before I started, down to the very last drop, which I acknowledged was the last drop. I felt more involved in right here and now. I felt my impatience had evaporated and I was no longer in such a hurry to go and grab some free food and speak to people. I felt satisfied mentally and physically, although I did notice I was still hungry.

Summary and tips:
Whether you just fill the mugs or do the full exercise of emptying them again, this is a great exercise for calming nerves and impatience. This is meditation with mugs. And it's extremely calming, like a euphoric opiate. The exercise put a smile on my face before lunch.

Day 15: 'Curiosity and self-forgiveness' (exercising tolerance of self)

It's Monday morning, two coffees into the day and the air temperature has defrosted enough for me to open the doors and let the sunshine in. My girlfriend and I had a frustrating telephone conversation about our frustrations about not being physically together, which led to feelings of regret about being here in Australia, and although I know I'm close to landing a job that will allow me to travel back to New York and to her, I can imagine for her in the US, it's harder having even less control over the physical separation than I do. Self-doubt has a tendency to creep into these moments, so what better a time than now to exercise some tolerance of myself.

I follow the instructions from *The Happiness Animal* and write down five sentences that begin with the words 'I notice':

I notice the pressure from my left shin on the back of my right ankle
I notice the feeling of my sock on the toes of my left foot.
I notice pressure of my laptop squashing my hand flesh against the base bone where my left hand meets my wrist.
I notice the sound of birds tweeting
I notice the sound of crickets

As I finish the above I begin to feel more focused and present again, less distracted, just as was the case in the previous exercise for patience and the exercise for connecting with words. All three of these exercises seem to bring about a relaxed and meditative feeling of wellness.

I continue this exercise by writing down five things that I imagine right now, but before I do, I realize that the exercise would have been better constructed if the imagining sentences came before the noticing. Now that I have noticed and feel grounded, I am finding it harder to imagine. But here goes:

I imagine I'm getting a headache.
I imagine I've been away from my girlfriend too long and she is likely to get tempted to cheat on me.
I imagine when she goes out with her younger friend that a lot of attractive men will talk to her, chat her up, and tempt her.
I imagine if she feels restricted that she can't be physical with other people, it will be my fault.
I imagine I won't get to New York until July.

I enter the numbers into the following sentences, per the exercise instructions:

1 thing I notice about myself (the squished hand on the laptop) is negative.
5 things I imagine about myself are negative.

I laugh when read I these sentences back. And I see my human predicament right in front of me. My life is pretty good 80% of the time when I use my senses, but 100% bad when I use my imagination to live. I laugh out loud at myself some more.

   After another coffee, I get started on the optional part II of the exercise for self-forgiveness: I take a blank piece of paper and write 'I can't forgive myself for…' at the top. Then as the exercise progresses (see appendix, page 139) I'm asked to write about the positive reasons why I did what I can't forgive myself for. I find one of the biggest revelations and something that gives me a feeling of reassurance and self-compassion, was the positive reason why I did something. Even though I felt self-compassion and a sense of calm for the negative reason why I did something, it was the positive that uplifted my spirit the most as I sat at the desk, writing on the blank piece of paper. I realize nothing is preventing me from forgiving myself now, which in itself makes it feel as if weight is lifted from my torso. I feel a general lightness and sense of being unburdened. I feel contentment with living a simple existence. Then I write a letter to myself from the perspective of a friend, who is the first person who springs to mind when I think of the word 'compassionate' and non-judgmental. I decide to call the friend and tell them I appreciate how compassionate they are. I feel less alone, more connected to my life, more awake, and oddly enough, I am getting pretty hungry.
   The exercise instructions say to put aside the letter that I have written from the perspective of the friend, and come back to it and read it again after a few days, so this is what I do. It's now Wednesday. I woke at 6am today, feeling a little cloudy headed despite two cups of coffee. I pull out the letter again, and even though I know I wrote it, I hear my friend's voice as I am reading the words and imagine it's her talking to me. I ask myself the following question: Am I more valuable to others as a vulnerable human being who is still willing to step into the arena, who is willing to dare to do better but who admits to making mistakes, or am I more valuable as someone who hides secrets, and poisons themselves with their own self-judgment and shame? And I feel confident about my answer and my conviction to be honest about who I am in this world. This confidence and conviction gives me an immediate sense of connection with the world.
   There is an optional further step to this exercise, which is to share my story. People like to know they are not alone in not being perfect. In this instance I share my story with my radical honesty friends on an email group we set up after a workshop in Greece. Once I have sent the email, I laugh

some more about my human predicament and feel more connected having just shared my human experience with a group of people whom I have been radically honest with in the past. Funnily enough, earlier this morning my girlfriend had opened up to me that sometimes she hides away from the world and I told her that I do the same. The flow of us sharing our thoughts and feelings on a similar experience connected us. Even though she's in the USA and I'm in Australia, I felt closer to her after that conversation.

Summary and tips:
This is an exercise for 'taking a load off'. After the exercise I feel a little tension in my stomach but comforted by the knowledge that all of my problems only exist as problems in my imagination, with the exception of physical discomforts like having too much pressure on my bony wrist. So it's time to take a break from typing.

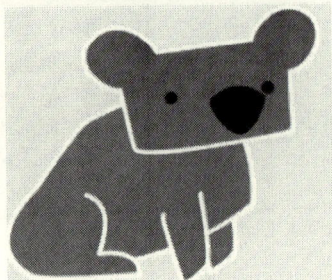

<u>Chapter 4</u>

Five days aware

It is not that we have a short time to live but that we waste a lot of it

They achieve what they want laboriously; they possess what they have achieved anxiously; and meanwhile they take no account of time that will never more return.
It is a small part of life that we really live.
Until we have begun to go without certain things, we fail to realize how unnecessary many things are. We have been using them not because we needed them but because we had them

Seneca

If you wish to enrich Pythocles, do not add to his riches, but lessen his desires

Epicurus

I lived a life of excesses and extremes. All in or all out. A great boyfriend or a crappy one. Drinking heavily or complete abstinence. The biggest bouquets of flowers, or no flowers at all. Lobster tails or baked beans. Very considerate or very inconsiderate. There was little in between. And little did I know I was no more in control of my life than a ball in a pinball machine. Until I began working on *The Happiness Animal*, my awareness of my susceptibility to attraction, distraction and desires was limited, as was my awareness of the source of my thoughts. I wasn't paying attention to what the impact on my happiness would be when my thinking links led me to their destination of desire. Once I started noticing with my senses what was happening and then seeing my thoughts for what they actually are – just thoughts created in my imagination – then I realized I could be the pinball player, and if I wanted to I didn't have to play the game at all. When I started noticing that I was imagining thoughts, and when I could see the thoughts I was imagining, and became aware that I didn't have to listen to my imagination and its self-justified thoughts, the '*it will help you calm down before you see Juliette. Just one,*' but that I could accept them for what they were, just thoughts, let them pass and use my senses instead, my life became instantly simpler, healthier and happier. Awareness is also an unhappiness preventer. If kindness, honesty, tolerance and courage do for your happiness what a blue (reliever) inhaler does for asthma, then awareness is both the blue and the brown (problem preventer). And unlike asthma medication, there are no side effects to using awareness. So let's suck it in…

Day 16: 'The tempting way to self-control' (exercising awareness with FAD (Food, Alcohol and other Drugs)

It's Friday, 1pm. I am feeling tension and a little malaise today. I received an email overnight informing me that I wouldn't be offered a job and that my visa status was a factor. I feel disappointed. I also feel under pressure as I attended a presentation last night to purchase timeshare accommodation on the premise that I'd receive two free gift cards for an Australian supermarket simply for attending, and today I will need to tell salesman I have changed my mind and can't afford it. I feel disconnected and demoralized for having misled the salesman into believing I would purchase the timeshare, even though I was aware of the psychology techniques the sales staff were employing to manipulate me into saying yes. I feel like going to the bar and ordering a beer, even though I know it isn't healthy for my body, nor my happiness, nor my authenticity. So it's a perfect time to exercise some awareness.

The first instruction is for me to pause. Then I complete the following steps:

1. Notice the sensations in your body associated with your feelings and thoughts compelling you to consume. What feelings (e.g. tension in my forehead) are you feeling in different parts of your body?

    Tension across the front of my belly, increased salivation, hunger, thirst tension in palate tongue pressed against palate, and clenched jaws. There is considerable tension in my cheeks and across my forehead.

2. What do you feel is your inadequacy? Try and define your source of feelings of inadequacy as specifically as possible. Are they sourced in fear of something? What are your thoughts associated with this fear?

    I feel my inadequacy is that I'm not good enough to get a job. My thoughts are about my lack of money, and my lack of connection with my girlfriend. They are thoughts of loneliness and of rejection. The underlying fear is that I will be isolated and alone without enough money to live. It's both a fear of being alone and a fear of not being able to live.

3. How do you feel consuming will help with this inadequacy?

    It may relax my head, reduce my fear, help me to forget.

4. Before you consume, ask yourself the following four questions:

    A. Will it bring me power of the genuine [internally authentic] sort?
    No

    B. Will it increase my level of enlightenment?
No, although it may relax me enough to have more thoughts other than those about the job and not having a concrete plan for getting back to my girlfriend. That, said, based on previous experience, it may increase my negative thoughts and make me feel depressed.

    C. Will it make me more whole?
No. It will numb my senses and make me less of me.

    D. Will it make me more loving?
No, based on previous experience, it will make me sleazy, not more loving.

5. Now notice with your senses what your body wants. If your muscles feel tired, it could be sleep. If your throat is dry, it could be water. If you have pressure in your bladder or your bowels, maybe you want to go to the toilet. Write it down here:

Need more warmth or clothing. Need to go to the bathroom, need to eat, dry throat, need to drink some water.

6. Is what you wrote down in step 5 different to what your mind wants you to consume? The secret to releasing yourself from excess is to start living from what you notice you want rather than what your mind says you should want.

Yes it is different.

7. Now go back and repeat step 2. Focus on the physical sensations you are having that your mind is associating with the compulsion to consume. Rate your level of pain or discomfort of not giving into the compulsion to consume on a level of 1-10 with 10 being intolerable agony and preferring to die.

8. Reality test your pain/discomfort. Can you live with it? Can you survive it?

Yes

9. Allow yourself to fully experience and notice those sensations now. The more you allow yourself to experience them, the more they will have been experienced fully and therefore disappear of their own accord. The alternative, which is resisting those sensations, allows those sensations to persist. The only way to ease them is to allow yourself to experience each physical sensation individually and to stop resisting its perceived unpleasantness. Your mind is a drama queen. The sensations are never as bad as you think they are. It helps if you notice when each sensation appears in your body and if you describe each sensation individually. Describe each sensation below now and then focus your attention on each in turn. Allow yourself to fully experience (and feel) each sensation.

Like a tight rubber band is around my crown, and like my stomach is an empty inflating balloon. As I write this down I notice the sensations diminishing. I feel more awake and my eyes actually feel refreshed.

****

About a month after the above exercise, I'd been to the thank you afternoon tea, which I talked about in the exercise for washing my words ('Call it bullshit'). One of the other attendees of the afternoon tea mentioned she was going to an experiential art installation by Marina Abramovic – an artist I literally stumbled on in New York when I happened to be walking past the opening night of one of her art installations. Abramovic's art, in my opinion, opens us up to new ways of experiencing what it is to be a human being and channels this experience by heightening our awareness through specific senses. Abramovic works with the idea that removing one or more of our senses heightens our remaining senses. Both installations I've been to required the wearing of soundproof headphones, and in New York, I also had to wear a blindfold. After I attended the Sydney installation, I was walking home past the bars and restaurants on Sydney harbor's waterfront, and I felt a real buzz in my head. I thought about going to a bar but didn't, remembering what happened last time I did that. Instead, I went back to the house and fed the husky. And then decided to have a double shot of my housemate's whisky. What I noticed was an immediate dulling of my senses that had been so sharp at Marina Abramovic. I felt like I'd taken painkillers and I was slow, wasn't able to think as quickly and had less control over the words coming out of my mouth when talking to my housemate's mother. I was louder. I had lost interest in checking train times for my next move. The dulling of my senses was replaced, as the alcohol left my system, with a mental tension like someone had painlessly inserted a giant, empty syringe into my forehead and was sucking fluid from my brain. I wanted to replace that fluid with alcohol. I felt the tension, the frown and repeated the exercise of focusing on the sensations I could notice in my body. I then watched a film with a cup of tea, went back to the sensations, then they diminished, but I'd lost my drive and energy for the day. So I went to bed. And slept. I'm writing this the next morning. I feel quite empowered and more in control, rather than controlled by addiction. But given I felt no benefits to drinking I have no desire to repeat this exercise again.

Summary and tips:
Discomfort or wanting to change my thoughts or how I'm feeling is better relieved by exercising awareness than by painkillers or alcohol. By accepting and noticing my thoughts, then contrasting that with noticing physical sensations in my body, I feel instantly grounded and no longer at the whim of those thoughts. By delimiting the discomfort that I want to rid myself of to physical sensations I can notice, and by paying attention to sensations, I am able to reduce the discomfort, rather than magnifying it in the abstraction and associations of my imagination.

Day 17: 'The conscious veto' (exercising awareness with doing)

It's Friday, 1:43 pm. This is only the second exercise so far that I'm starting after lunch. On a day with a lot of uncertainty around a job application I currently have in progress and uncertainty around when I can travel back to the USA, I've been trying and failing to complete tasks on my to-do list. The wind outside is strong and cold. I have had the fire lit all morning and had one less coffee than normal. The heat haze from the fire, consuming oxygen out of the room and the lack of fresh air are contributing, I imagine, to me feeling somewhat spaced out and frustrated with not being able to book a flight, while knowing that there is a flight sale on at the moment which will end on Monday. A state of having things to do and being frustrated with not being able to do them is a perfect opportunity for this exercise...

The first step is for me to look my to-do list, which I have scribbled inside my moleskin notebook. Then I classify my tasks as follows:

- Mark only those items that are an absolute necessity to me and my family staying alive with an '**N**' for necessity.
- Mark the things I think I should do with an '**S**' for SHIT (one of the golden rules in *The Happiness Animal* is that when I should on myself, I shit on myself. Shitting on myself is fairly demoralizing).
- Mark those things I genuinely want to do with a '**W**' for want.

I found that some of the items I would have said 'I need to do' were not an absolute necessity to me staying alive. The truth was more that I preferred (wanted) to do them, and less that I actually needed to do them. Putting a 'W' next to items that I had considered a necessity, which weren't actually, changed my feelings towards the tasks away from discomfort and avoidance and I noticed my forehead relaxing when I added the 'W'. Now that these items were no longer a true necessity but something I actually wanted to do, I wasn't dreading the phone call with the HR manager. Instead I *wanted* to call him to seek a solution. The final classifications for my to-do list today are as follows: N: 0; W: 31; S: 7. As I went through the list, it also prompted me to act on some quick wins: I sent a couple of emails, made a phone call and these quick actions resulted in a some of the 'W' tasks being completed and crossed off the list. I could book that train ticket from Sydney to Canberra now that I knew when I'd be travelling. Per the exercise instructions I also choose some of the S's to veto and cross off my list. I vetoed five out of the seven S's which equates to about a 15% reduction in my overall to-do list. I feel encouraged that most of what is left in my list is things I want to do (or would prefer I do rather than not do). The list also feels tighter and more meaningful now I have scratched the 15% shit out of it!

The next instruction is to practice doing the following for the next week: every time I have a thought to do something, ask myself if it is something I want or need to do. If it isn't, veto it. If I can notice the origin of the thought, I ask myself what previous thoughts caused me to have that thought? I need to be aware that I am noticing myself having the thought to do whatever it is, and I am consciously choosing to veto it.

Part II of the exercise, is to go on a choice diet. Today the choices for which I will limit the amount of time or number of options I'll consider are: Looking at flight options. I decide to cut off my flight browsing for the day and make my decision confidently that I won't book a flight until I have a job offer (rather than going onto the flight search websites every day for a look). By making a firm decision, even though it is of no great consequence, I feel instantly more grounded and less doubtful of my actions as I land below the clouds of indecision. I feel sharper and the woozy feeling I've been having today is subsiding. I feel more alert and awake despite having missed my regular third coffee of the day. I decide to stick to two coffees and not make a third. Great. No more second guessing…

Summary and tips:
Sometimes I have a tendency to overanalyze and procrastinate rather than make a decision. Often, especially when the decision is of no great consequence (what item to choose off a menu), it's less demoralizing to make a 'wrong' decision than to procrastinate. Making decisions, and eliminating the unnecessary items in my to do list, creates head space, that gives me a sense of greater control over my life, and allows me the time and space to relax. It also offers me the space to remain a conscious noticer of my thoughts rather than get carried away by my thinking links that more often than not lead to demoralizing destinations.

Day 18: 'Time isn't money and money isn't time' (exercising awareness of time and money)

It's Monday morning, again at the frosty lake house, two coffees in at 9am. Later today I will plant some organic garlic, something I have been helping the neighboring German farmers with for a couple of days now, and for which they pay me a generous salary of twenty dollars an hour. But right now, as I look at the title of the exercise I am going to use to strengthen my happiness today, my thoughts form a philosophical exploration that culminates in me writing in my notebook: *Time is no more than a series of*

uniform and consistent movements. The word movements seems to resonate in my gut. I continue writing…
Do you want to measure your life in the currency of uniform and consistent movements?
My answer is almost certainly no. I continue….
But all those quantities of movements are taking place in the infinite plane of the present.
And then an afterthought…
There is more life in movement than in money, but not in the uniform kind.

It feels like this monologue offers an insight into my attitude towards both time and money as I begin this exercise.

Part I of the exercise is for identifying what is enough when it comes to work and money. As I write my answers to the exercise questions below, I feel some minor tension across the front of my belly...

1. How many hours of work would you like to accomplish in a working week? **Tip**: if it's over 40 you may have a problem

    14

    I chuckled as I wrote this. Two hours per day of the week feels like a good balance. I feel I do two hours of really focused, quality work per day and then my attention isn't as of such high quality.

2. What do you consider to be enough hours for you to work a week?

    10

    I chuckled as I wrote this too. I decided to give myself the weekend off.

3. How many activities would you like to accomplish in a week in addition to your work?

    14

    Before I wrote this, I checked my to-do list (some of the activities in the list are work related but I wouldn't classify as work given I don't feel a sense of obligation, but more a sense of wanting to do them for my own benefit). Then I changed my mind about checking the to-do list and felt that it'd be great if I could accomplish two activities in addition to work each day.

4. How many hours would a week do you want to spend on those activities?

_____14_____

5. How much money do you want to earn as a minimum in a working week?

_____$700_____

6. What do you consider enough money for you to earn in a working week? **Tip**: once you cover basic needs (estimated at $40000 USD a year in the USA) any increase in your cash levels will not have an impact on your happiness

_____$700_____

My first instinct was to put $500 for question five and six. $500 a week felt like enough for both, although I imagine that feeling may quickly change as soon as I get back to living in Manhattan. The reality is that for the next twelve months I plan to get a job that pays $90,000 gross a year and supplement that income with Airbnb income, until I am able to live off Airbnb income and book royalties. As soon as I commit to a full time job for the near future, my expectations of money per week immediately go up. But in my current enjoyable lifestyle of house-sitting and looking after pets and writing, $500 a week is more than enough. It's only when I start planning for the future that I start thinking about larger amounts, and I notice that when I do so, my mood instantly lowers, and my forehead furrows with tension. I also feel the tension in my stomach. So I'd prefer to stick to the present for now and forget my high (salary) expectations of the future. Part II of the exercise is designed to help with exactly that, getting back to the present, whenever I feel dominated by thoughts of money or all the things I still have to do at work. This also works as a relaxation and grounding-in-the-present-moment technique for any scenario. Per the exercise, I focus on becoming conscious of the feeling of the air going in and out of my body as I breathe. This instantly relaxes my shoulders, my stomach and brings a sense of general comfort and ease. I notice there is about a two and a half second pause in between the end of my in breath and the beginning of my out breath.

I notice there is about a four second pause in between the end of my out breath and the beginning of my in breath. Now I'm starting to feel a sleepy. I repeat the noticing of the breath pause durations for about four breaths. The more I notice the pauses in between breaths, the more I notice myself feeling more awake again, but the calmness remains. I'm ready to get to work and plant some garlic.

Summary and tips:
I will be honest and say that I didn't feel a major impact to my happiness doing Part I of this exercise. In fact, focusing attention on money was somewhat demoralizing and uncomfortable for me. Perhaps that is due to my apprehension and associated tension from what I think about returning to the workforce. Then I realize all I have to do is stay true to how I feel and express myself honestly when I go back to work. I can survive the worst that can happen in the workplace so I might as well relax, and enjoy experiencing the experience of work in New York City. This exercise did also help me to reality test what is enough and notice that I am striving for more than what is enough. Perhaps that awareness is enough.

Day 19: 'The tempting way to self-control II' (exercising awareness of desire)

It's Saturday, my last Saturday at the lake house. I'm tired, a little groggy today, probably from travelling to Sydney two days ago for training for the 'Happiness and its Causes' conference, sleeping at an Airbnb and then coming back yesterday on the train. My former housemate, with whom I had become intimate with on several occasions, had asked if she could pay me a visit, and offered to give me a lift back to Sydney. Initially my thought had been that this would be fine. She could come and stay in the spare room on Tuesday night after going for a walk around in nature and then I could get a lift back to Sydney with her on Wednesday. In the last couple of days as her arrival would draw nearer though, I had both flashbacks to the past and thoughts I imagined of potential scenes that may come up were she to come here. Especially today. Staying in the same house at night, the wood fire, imagining that it would be possible for her dress provocatively or while walking through the house after taking a shower, I imagined that the opportunity for intended or unintended seduction could arise and my relaxed feeling of ease with life and enjoyment of the moment that I had been experiencing up until this morning was replaced by a demoralizing feeling of discomfort in my stomach and across my head. I realized my gut was telling me it was a bad idea for her to come. I loved my girlfriend and didn't want to do anything to risk damaging my relationship with her. While I had a compulsive desire to receive some human company after spending a month pretty much alone in the country, I knew deep down that it wouldn't be healthy for my relationship with my girlfriend or my happiness. And so, it was a perfect time for me to pull this exercise up on my girlfriend's laptop...

The first instruction of the exercise is to accept that I am attracted to other people other than my partner. If the other person is flirting with me or making physical (sexual) advances towards me, I need to communicate to this person that I want to respect my love of my girlfriend. So I decide to write an email to the former housemate, and tell her not to come. I tell her that I am not comfortable with her being physically present here. I also am asked to complete the following questions which I have answered below.

1. Notice the sensations in your body associated with your feelings compelling you to cheat. What feelings (e.g. tension) are you feeling in different parts of your body?

   Not compelled to cheat, but I feel tension in my stomach, as if it is caving inwards, tension in my head (almost a mild headache), clenched jaw.

2. What do you feel is your inadequacy? Try and define your source of feelings of inadequacy as specifically as possible. Are they sourced in a feeling that you are not getting enough attention/affection from your current partner? Is it that you don't feel you can communicate fully with your partner? When was the last time YOU initiated an open and honest conversation with your partner?

   It is a feeling of loneliness and wanting physical affection from my partner who is in New York. The last time I initiated an open and honest conversation with my partner was a few days ago, so I tell her how I'm feeling now.

3. How do you feel cheating on your partner will help with this inadequacy?

It will not but communicating honestly with my girlfriend about how much I am craving her affection has already helped.

4. Before you cheat, ask yourself the following four questions:

   a. Will it bring me power of the genuine [internally authentic] sort?
   No

   b. Will it increase my level of enlightenment?
   No

   c. Will it make me more whole?
   No

   d. Will it make me more loving?
   No

5. Now notice with your senses what your body wants. If your muscles feel tired, it could be sleep. If your throat is dry, it could be water. If you have pressure in your bladder or your bowels, maybe you want to go to the toilet. Write it down here:

Sleep. Water. A shower or bath. Some food. Sex.

Being able to get specific about what my body and my soul want (intimacy with my girlfriend and a strong physical and honest connection with her) transforms me into being clear and confident about my actions. I feel pressure has been lifted from my body. While I had still been open to the idea of allowing the former housemate to stay in the spare room, I felt boxed into a corner of a dark room in my head. I felt anxious. Now I feel free again, looking forward to enjoying the rest of the day outside in the sunshine and then inside with the view. Quite simply, I realized what my ego wanted (attention) is not what I want. It is not what I want in a physical, intimate sense from anyone other than my girlfriend. Articulating it specifically has helped me to know what I do want. And being able to trust my own wants as a guide for what is healthy for my happiness is a huge relief. I can relax.

Summary and tips:
You don't need to be contemplating cheating to do this exercise. It can be used in situations where if you met up with someone or spent time with them, your gut feeling would make you uncomfortable.

Day 20: 'How to stop shitting on myself' (exercising awareness with conformity and moralizing)

It's Tuesday morning in the Australian countryside, still Monday night of Memorial Day in the USA. I received some personal criticism from a former housemate by email this morning, which I responded to with my own specific resentment directed at them. I also had a mix up with my iPhone, which I had sold on eBay: the auction winner hadn't responded or paid so I offered the next highest bidder a 'second chance offer'. Now I have received two payments for one item and have a dilemma on who I should (with the emphasis on should) give the phone to. Then I realize the best I can do is be honest to both sellers about the situation and ask them what would be the best thing to do. I feel instantly less tension as soon as I seek their input. But the situation does provide me with a useful example where I catch myself shoulding (or shitting on) myself. That's exactly what the following exercise is for and I'm smiling as I write this. I had a lot of fun with talking about shoulding and shitting during my public talk in New York last November, and with my coaching clients. This exercise is also something that I imagine would be fun at a house party...

The exercise is for me to replace the word 'toilet' with the word 'should' so the first thing I'm going to do, with a smile and a giggle, is to take a piece of paper and write 'should' on it and put it up on the toilet door. The next thing I do is write 'Should Shit Log' (SSL) 26th May – 2nd June 2015 on the top of a page in my notebook. Every time I notice myself saying the word 'should' for the next week, I'm going to write it down in that notebook and replace the word 'should' with the word 'shit'. I will add my entries in here after I'm done (see page 72). The next part of the exercise instructs me to write down my favorite limiting beliefs that I impose on my existence, and for every limiting belief I write down 'I squirt shit on myself' in my Should Shit Log (SSL). Here are mine:

I squirt shit on myself. I don't know enough about markets to work for Reuters.

I squirt shit on myself. I don't have enough money to get married.

I squirt shit on myself. My book hasn't sold enough copies for people to take me seriously as a happiness speaker.

I squirt shit on myself. I've been out of work too long for a company to give me a job.

I squirt shit on myself. I don't have enough charisma to interest people in what I have to say.

I squirt shit on myself. I'm too stupid to work in an office and use their processes.

As I write, I think and speak the specifics of each thought out loud and I realize both how ridiculous my own imagined obstacles are and how easily they can be overcome – that is if the obstacles actually exist in reality at all. I laugh an out breath and smile. My limiting beliefs seem a lot smaller on paper than in my head. I need to stop squirting on myself and the first step is becoming more aware of when I'm doing it. Making an entry in my Should Shit Log every time I squirt shit on myself over the following week will exercise that awareness.

The next part of the exercise is writing down how I normally shoot myself in the foot. Every time I shoot myself in the foot I will write 'I constipate myself' in my Should Shit Log. But before I even get started with that, I can already think of the following constipations...

I constipate myself by browsing Facebook and Twitter.

I constipate myself by browsing the internet.

I constipate myself by checking email inboxes.

I constipate myself with impatience and wanting to make plans for the future now.

$$*****$$

For those of you who are interested, here is my Should Shit Log for the week where, every time I caught myself using the word 'should' I replaced it with 'shit':

26th May: *I shit on myself to change the exercise for 'Time isn't money' into something that has more of a direct impact on happiness.*

26th May: *How students shit, I shit on students on how to respond to an article.*

27h May: *You shit, I shit on you.*

27th May: *You shit, I shit on you to go get it first.*

27th May: *You shit, I shit on you to be inside in the morning, outside in the afternoon.*

27th May: *I shit on myself to write a children's book version of The Happiness Animal.*

28th May: *I shit on myself to eat something*

28th May: *You shit, I shit on you to only do something if you want to.*

29th May: *I shit on myself to have bought a bottle of water.*

29th May: *I shit on myself to finish the book soon.*

30th May: *How long do you think I shit on myself wait before contacting them?*

Thankfully the frequency of shitting on myself dropped off after the first three to four days, just as anyone would be put off from eating an unpleasant food after the first few tries. The only thing left for me to do is to flush my Should Shit Log down the toilet.

Summary and tips:
Throughout the course of the week I've become more aware of how often I shit on myself (squirting or otherwise) or constipate myself with limiting beliefs. I've chuckled with others and brought the concept of the Should Shit Log up in conversation. I decided to leave the 'should' sign up on the toilet door so that when my friends return to their house it will provoke them into healthy curiosity. The exercise made me an objective observer of the language I'm using to both speak and think with, and has helped me tweak my choice of words in favor of my own happiness. Choosing my words can be a lot of fun, and helps connect me to others by expressing what I truly feel, not what I should.

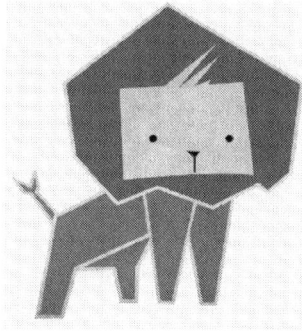

Chapter 5

Five days courageous

There is nothing fearful except fear itself. It is not that we have fears in the daylight but that we have entirely created darkness for ourselves. If you can look directly at things they often cease to be frightening

It is not because things are hard that we lack confidence but things are hard because we lack the confidence in the first place

Seneca

Creating is the place where the human spirit shines its brightest light

Robert Fritz

Before I was deep into writing *The Happiness Animal*, shirking, hiding, and avoiding social situations were common behaviors for me. If I could get out of a work meeting, I'd make it happen. Anything but having to interact with other people who, I imagined, would be judging me constantly. *Am I using the right acronym? Can that manager notice that there's a bead of sweat coming through my shirt? Does my voice sound monotonous? Do they hate me? Do I look scruffy? Do I sound stupid?* Outside of work, when I gave up drinking I felt like a social pariah, like I had some kind of infectious disease I had to hide. I imagined that other people thought I was abnormal, retarded or something. That everything said I was dumb. Stupid. That I was an embarrassment to the group, and by association, to the entire human race. Like that socially illiterate, uncool country cousin you wouldn't want your cool city friends to meet. No mojo, street stupid, blunt. I felt awkward, uncomfortable, my voice muffled and strained when I spoke so that people in the bar couldn't hear me properly. I lost my voice, or I hadn't yet found it. I strained under the tension of my torso and my head, my shoulders raised, to think of something to say to join in the conversation and to feel at ease, but I felt like an alien who had nothing to offer the tomfoolery of the situation. That was, unless I drank. I avoided my friend's party because I had fear of being judged, fear I wasn't cool enough for the conversation, fear that I wouldn't fit in. Little did I realize at the time, this was an incredibly self-centered view. The irony of my shyness and social anxiety was that I had it because I imagined that I was the centre of everyone's attention. A lot of reality testing later, now I relish opportunities to meet new people and to expose myself socially. If I can open a new connection to the world through someone else, I will. I also enjoy deepening my existing connections. But I can usually do with a little extra courage socially to prevent me from slipping back into my own self-centered thinking. Having some courage can be extremely useful when it comes to being myself and speaking my authentic view socially, but with the exercises that follow I'm excited to be taking courage a step further along the path of fearlessness. I'm ready to face my fears.

Day 21: 'What am I afraid of?' (exercising acceptance of fear)

On day eleven, I exercised tolerance of my fear and anxiety relating to my liver, and reality-tested my imagination. If that was an exercise in tolerance and reality-testing, today is an exercise in awareness and acceptance. This exercise is about becoming aware of all my fears and accepting them so that fears stop silently and subconsciously influencing me with me having no more control over them than I have control over the content of my dreams. By accepting that the fears are my fears just as my dreams are my dreams, I can choose to not let them influence my life while I am awake. The first part of this exercise requires me to make a list of my fears, so here it is:

Name of fear: Fear of losing money.

> **I notice these sensations with the fear:** It's a hollow feeling in my stomach and like reflux is coming into my throat.

> **Root of fear:** Fear of not being able to survive without money. – fear of dying.

Name of fear: Fear of not having a job.

> **I notice these sensations with the fear:** It's a feeling of someone squeezing the front of my head.

> **Root of fear:** Fear of not being able to survive without money. – fear of dying.

Name of fear: Fear of illness

> **I notice these sensations with the fear:** dryness on the sides of my tongue, slight salty taste in my mouth. Feeling of inflation inside my belly. Heat inside the lower half of my torso.

> **Root of fear:** Fear of disease/major illness.

> - fear of dying.

Name of fear: Fear of punishment (for not paying bills)

I notice these sensations with the fear: constriction in my throat, my stomach, across my shoulders. General tension in my face.

Root of fear: Fear of fines, of being imprisoned.

- fear of losing freedom.

The next instruction is to go back and read my fears one by one, and notice the feelings I associate with my fear again. The instruction is to stick with the sensations, noticing the specifics in my body without trying to diminish or avoid them, but to accept them and be aware of them. So I spend a couple of minutes focusing on experiencing each bodily sensation. The more I read my sensations and focus on my fears, the more insignificant and abstract they seem. They don't feel connected to me and are more just thoughts on paper. It feels like I'm untangled from them, and freer. I feel less afraid now I have been able to articulate very specifically what it is I am afraid of. Instead of being a large looming and vague intangible darkness, my fear has been delimited to four simple things. I'm feeling more relaxed, clear headed and calm.

Summary and tips:

This exercise can be done in a couple of minutes, yet it can be a grounding and confidence building technique that can be used in any situation of vague uncertainty, anxiety or fear. Once I'm aware of what specifically it is that I fear, I can accept it, notice how that fear translates into physical sensations that I can pinpoint in my body, and the fear ceases to dominate me. It's fear, delimited.

Day 22: 'Choosing the unknown' (exercising courage with the unknown)

This is an exercise I am choosing to do deliberately when I feel most alone and most uncertain of the future. For me that emotion normally comes about when I am physically alone and after dark. But today it's Sunday, I have some kind of cold or flu. I've just had lunch alone, it's been raining outside, I still don't have a job, and the house I'm in is cold. I have a strange taste in my mouth. I'm worried my past excessive drinking has damaged my kidneys and liver. I'm worried about dying young. My closest friend in Australia is about to leave the country and go back to France. I don't know how I will fund my trip back to New York. It is uncertain whether I will be able to take out money from my pension fund early, and if I can't I will have to borrow money from my parents, or not go to New York at all. I'd either be stranded here, alone in Australia, or go back to my parent's farm in Cornwall as a seemingly useless job-reject, filled with a feeling of unworthiness and shame. My current poor health makes me feel impotent and I even worry that I won't be physically man enough to satisfy my girlfriend in the bedroom if I do make it back to New York. I can't think of a better day to exercise courage with the unknown. This exercise for facing uncertainty, the unknown and emptiness is meant to be done before I go to sleep so I may have a siesta this afternoon and do it now. I lay down in bed, after closing the blinds.

The instructions are to close my eyes for fifteen minutes and do the following:

1. Focus on a feeling of emptiness while my eyes are closed.

2. Focus on falling deeper and deeper into my emptiness.

3. Accept the emptiness. Let it be there inside of me or all around me.

4. If fear arises – let that be there too. Notice the feeling of my fear and stay focused on noticing the emptiness.

5. I may tremble with fear but I am not to reject this space that is being born there in the emptiness.

I followed the instructions. At first I began by lying on my back, but then I found it hard to imagine falling into emptiness. So then I lay face down into a pillow. I was surrounded by blackness, felt the falling sensation, felt a little fear, I imagined my body became just an outline filled with empty space and I was just empty space. Flashes of fear darted into the experience. Occasional shapes formed in the emptiness and a little white light came and went, morphing forms from faces to animals swallowing. After a while in the darkness and accepting my hollow outline I became comfortable with the nothingness of everything. My fears concerning my physical health disappeared. I became a little sexually aroused. And then I went to sleep for about thirty minutes. I am now writing this at 4pm, with a mug of green tea, feeling like I have awakened from a deep, deep sleep. Refreshed, yet still bleary eyed, somehow cleansed, and healthier. My negative thinking links feel broken. It feels like a new morning. The feeling you get when you get out of hospital after a few days. I feel unburdened from worries and anxieties. Just awake.

*****

Summary and tips:
It's now a couple of days later and this exercise is now my go to strategy for any kind of anxieties or fears related to my health. I find I only need to focus on the feeling of emptiness for a couple of minutes with my eyes closed to get the same benefits that took about 15 minutes the first time.

Day 23: 'Finding my signature talent' (exercising courage with action)

This Sunday morning I have been feeling a little disconnected. It's now been over a month since I've been living alone in the lake house and I'm still waiting to hear about whether I will be offered a job or in New York. It's been three months since I last saw my girlfriend and five months since I saw my family. I have been thinking about the logistics of cleaning this house and getting to Sydney this coming Wednesday. So yes, as I have been thinking about the future I haven't been entirely present this morning. I'm somewhat adrift in a sea of uncertainty. Fortunately there is no better navigation tool for this sea than today's exercise...

If you are like me, being asked what your talents are can be a difficult question to answer. Too abstract to answer with specifics. The point of knowing what my talents are is that I can choose to do things in life which allow me to make use of my strengths, and in a way that I maximize how much of my talent I contribute to the world. This will ideally strengthen my connection to society and give me a greater sense of belonging and usefulness in that society. One of my disbeliefs growing up, and in working life was that I was 'useless'. In the past, this belief has sapped my social confidence, to the point of me avoiding social events. I alienated myself from others and felt disconnected. I did not belong in this world for as long as I was useless to this world. This belief can spiral quickly into depression. It is important then for me to exercise regularly to be regularly reminded of what my signature talent is. Knowing my signature talent gives me the courage to act in situations where I know I have the talent.

The first part of the exercise requires me to take Dr Martin Seligman's VIA 'Signature Strengths Test'. For me, Seligman is the Godfather of Positive Psychology and still runs a Masters course in Applied Positive Psychology at the University of Pennsylvania. I click on this link https://www.authentichappiness.sas.upenn.edu/testcenter and find the test. I find a temptation to answer some questions as I'd like the answers to be, rather than how things are. I break the 240 questions up with cups of tea, small chores and come back and do another 20 questions. All up it took me about 45 minutes to complete. And then came the results screen:

Your Top strength:

Forgiveness and mercy -

You forgive those who have done you wrong. You always give people a second chance. Your guiding principle is mercy and not revenge.

Interestingly the last time I took this test was 18 months ago and at the time my signature strength was my now number 3 strength...

Strength #3:

Creativity, ingenuity, and originality -

Thinking of new ways to do things is a crucial part of who you are. You are never content with doing something the conventional way if a better way is possible.

18 months ago I was still developing the original concepts for *The Happiness Animal*, whereas now I am working with my own existing model, so I agree that I am exhibiting less creativity today than I was 18 months ago. But I am exhibiting more forgiveness and mercy than I was 18 months ago: When I coach and help friends, I have become well practiced at not judging or blaming individuals, understanding the dynamics of the individual's situation, and that there are almost always thinking links and associations in play due to that individual's education of life. I do forgive easily, I am very much against the death penalty and am a big advocate of mercy.

The next part of the exercise is for me to identify which of my Happiness Animal's muscles corresponds to my top strength. Forgiveness and mercy are intrinsically both linked to tolerance and kindness. Next I am instructed to create a designated time in my schedule when I will exercise my top signature strengths (and corresponding happiness animal muscles) in a new way either inside or outside the workplace, by creating a clearly defined opportunity to use them. My second strength was assessed as:

Strength #2:

Fairness, equity, and justice -

Treating all people fairly is one of your abiding principles. You do not let your personal feelings bias your decisions about other people. You give everyone a chance.

So I try to think of a specific action I can take that combines forgiveness, mercy, fairness, equity and justice, and exercises my tolerance and kindness muscles. The first idea that pops into my head is that I could find out how to write a letter of compassion and forgiveness to a prisoner. So I write in my to-do list, *research ways to write letters to prisoners, identify one name and address and send a letter.* Imagining myself writing a letter to an inmate has already sparked new energy in me. I was feeling pretty lethargic right before this step of the exercise and was considering an early third coffee of the day. But now I have renewed enthusiasm for the day. I am feeling more awake, less tense and in a heightened mood or spirit. I will come back to this exercise to complete the remaining steps once I have engaged in the activity.

****

So it's been just over two months since I was last here. I have left the lake house. Here are the questions and my answers that complete the remainder of this exercise:

1. How did you feel before engaging in the activity of using your signature strength?

   Committed and confident, but I actually didn't write to the prisoner. Instead I wrote to an ex-girlfriend who owes me $1000 and a now valuable painting. I lent the money to her three years ago and she promised to pay me back. At the time she said I was a 'lifesaver'. At the moment, my finances are at the most depleted they've ever been given I quit my full-time job four years ago to become a dedicated writer. I need the money. The painting, by my godfather's father, was given to me by my parents when I was eighteen years old and holds both sentimental and financial value. The ex-girlfriend had agreed to look after this for me while I was travelling and keep it in 'a very safe place'. Now she says she hasn't been able to find it. Nor has she replied to my request for her to start paying me back. Prior to doing this exercise, I thought about taking her to the small claims court and sent her a text saying that if I hadn't her from her by the end of the week before last, I would have no other choice than the legal route. I felt a little demoralized after using the words 'small claims court'. It didn't feel right in my gut and the language I used felt threatening. So a week later I've decided to exercise some mercy, fairness, justice and forgiveness with her, and somehow fit all those strengths into one message. Here's the message:

Hi, have you worked out how much you can afford to pay back each fortnight from the $1000 I lent you in 2012?
When I thought about it, the small claims court doesn't feel right. So I won't do that. But I am in a tight spot financially and you did say you would pay me back. So I'm asking for you to be fair and reasonable. I know you can be both. I think if you can start paying me back say twenty dollars a fortnight, that's fair. And one day hopefully you will remember the very safe place you said you had put my painting in. All the best, Will

2. How did you feel during the activity?

A little fearful, but truthful, connected to what I was saying, empowered. Grounded in the present.

3. How did you feel after the activity?

Relieved.

4. Was the activity challenging or easy?

Challenging.

5. Did time pass quickly? Did you lose your sense of self-consciousness?

Yes. While I was focused on being non-judgmental, non–attacking and non-personal but simply asking for an action to take place now, rather than digging the past back up again and blaming.

6. Do you plan to repeat the exercise?

Yes

Day 24: 'Choose love' (exercising the courage to love)

Before I even attempt to begin today's exercise I've found a quote in the envelope pocket at the back of my notebook. The quote, on a small slip of green paper is something I had picked up from floor of the lake house south of Canberra. It was upside down on the floor and I thought it was just a piece of scrap for putting onto the fire, but when I turned it over and read it, it had a powerful and direct resonance. The quote reads: 'The deepest happiness you can have comes for that capacity to relieve the suffering of others'. While this might be a perfect quote to open the day of exercising compassion, I feel the resonance is even greater with the feeling of love. Given this is an exercise for loving the world and increasing your vulnerability, I'm using this quote here. As I write this, I am accompanied by a Siberian Husky dog. I'm sitting with a coffee at the café in Tamarama beach in Sydney. The instructions for the exercise are to pick something or someone to protect each day. Protecting Sierra (the husky) seems a little too easy but it is an accessible and achievable way for me to exercise. So I will give it a go, by ensuring she has enough water and food, and stops and sits at traffic lights.

*****

It was my job to protect the husky dog so I didn't get as much of a connection boost from what was already part of my routine and responsibility. But if I see a bug in the toilet, struggling to escape, I fish it out with some rolled up toilet paper rather than flushing it, and then I flick it off outside. If I see a caterpillar crossing the road, I pick it up and throw it in the hedge. Protecting even a small insect gives me an instant connection boost to the present moment. I feel useful, awake – like a haze has cleared from eyes – and more composed and grounded. Relaxed and confident. 'Trust and confidence' was voted the best definition of happiness in a global poll I ran for *The Happiness Animal* and it feels like this definition is not far off the mark.

The second part of the exercise is a little more directly achievable and can be accomplished in one go. It is to write a letter, opening up to someone I am close or intimate with about my greatest fears and my feelings for them. So I begin writing this letter now...

Dear Gina,

I want you to know that whenever I think of you, which is often, you bring a feeling of strength to my heart. A motivation not to give up in my pursuit of setting up a new life with you, in a new world. I feel love from my stomach to the top of my head and it makes my ears tingle. My greatest fear is that I wouldn't see you again, that I am not good enough, whatever that means, to get a job in New York, that I won't earn any money and that I won't be able to afford to live there with you. My greatest fear is that I will give up trying to work in New York, that my body will not be healthy enough, that my brain will not be strong enough. But then I look at your photograph, and I look at your smile, or I hear your voice on the telephone and I know that with patience and with persistence and with creative attempts, I will succeed beyond my expectations. I love you. I want to share experiences, share feelings and share my life with you. You bring warmth to the coldest bones in my body. You fill me with energy and with life, with strength, with courage, and with love. I love you Gina, and I'm so glad I asked you for directions two years ago in a bookstore in Denver.

Will

Expressing my fears to my girlfriend unburdened me, without even having to send the letter. My fears were no longer a heavy silent secret that just I was carrying around. Writing these fears also relieved some of the tension in my body and helped me to relax.

Summary and tips:
When I chose to protect something that was something I could have just as easily ignored, that is when I felt the benefits of this exercise the most, like

warmth flowing from my solar plexus. For the second part of the exercise, writing the letter to my girlfriend also renewed my appreciation for our relationship. Even reading the letter again now renews that appreciation. The letter also helped delimit my fears from the vague and uncertain to the specific. As I write this almost six months after the exercise, it also turns out my fears were unfounded: I now have a job in New York and am living with my girlfriend. Perhaps now I will show her the letter...

Day 25: 'Create my life' (exercising the courage to create)

It's Saturday, end of the morning, and by unforeseen circumstance I find myself back at the lake house, sitting outside at a table. I was up till 4am last night, trying to call potential employers in the USA and chatting online with my girlfriend. I am feeling tired, tense around my eyes and forehead and generally dirty on the inside, like I'm filled with a membrane of grime. I'm little flat after getting my hopes up about a job which it looked like I was being offered, until the company took a no-to-visas stance and blew me off. Still without a full-time paid job, I was able to do a lunchtime personal training for happiness session with a former colleague, to help them get specific and get over some workplace jealousy issues yesterday. And the two days prior I was working at the Happiness and its causes, world happiness conference attended by the Dalai Lama and sharing ideas with happiness experts, psychologists, and authors. I participated in dialogue that sparked some evolution of ideas on a subject that you can probably guess I am passionate about. Between my inner conflict of desperately seeking employment in the USA to ensure my speedy recovery to my girlfriend, and my passion for the study and practice of the best the world of happiness research has to offer, I can't think of a better time to exercise some creating using the courage of implementing my life purpose. Here's the exercise and my responses...

1. Below, list fifteen characteristics of your self. You may have previously considered some of them to be negative, but you can transform them in developing your life purpose. You may be intelligent, humorous, joyful, driven, slovenly, weird, whatever.

1____curious_____   6_____kind_____

2_____romantic_____   7_____honest_____

3_____sleazy_____   8____tolerant_____

4_____adaptive_____   9_____aware_____

5_____persistent_____   10_____ambitious_____

6_____resilient_____   11_____daring_____

7_____corny_____   12_____thoughtful_____

8_____shy_____   13_____considerate___

14_____loving_____   15_____addictive_____

If you didn't put fifteen down, get back up there and finish!

2. Now circle your five favorite personality characteristics. Do it quickly – don't think too much, or your ego will start to take over.

    I circled: Curious, kind, daring, loving and aware.

3. Referring loosely to the five favorite personality characteristics you just circled, make a list of fifteen actual behaviors that are ways you enjoy expressing these characteristics. For example, if one of your characteristics was generosity, then the behavior you perform in the real world that exemplifies generosity could be 'feeding the homeless by working in a soup kitchen on Sunday mornings'.

    a) Not taking 'no' for an answer, continuing to persist in finding solutions to obstacles and not giving up.

    b) Exercising awareness of how my thoughts influence my mood and ability to name my thoughts for what they are.

    c) Noticing when I can be assistance to others with small, everyday interactions and acting to help e.g. offering to carry bags.

d) Being affectionate and expressing love to the people I love.

e) Being my own psychologist to help myself out with negative thinking.

f) Continuing to ask questions on subjects that interest me like happiness. Not stopping with questions until my curiosity is satisfied.

g) Using my awareness in conversation and coaching to increase overall awareness in dialogue, helping others realize how they are thinking, and how their words are affecting their thoughts, their interpretations and associations with events, people and relationships.

At this point in the exercise I'm suffering from a little brain fog. It's also lunchtime (2:09 pm) and I decide to call it quits today and come back and finish this tomorrow with fresh eyes.

*****

OK I'm back.

h) Helping people resolve relationship and workplace problems with kindness, honesty, courage, awareness, curiosity and tolerance in my conversations with them.

i) Daring to do the things I enjoy in the workplace. Bringing the subject of happiness into the workplace.

j) Going on mini adventures like taking an inflatable kayak out to a remote stretch of river in the Australian bush (which I will do today), or crossing the Himalayas highest road pass solo on a motorbike.

k) Moving to a new location to be with my girlfriend, visiting family as often as possible. Hugging them all.

l) **Troubleshooting at work to find the right people who can fix the problem and eliminating problems (being a fixer).**

m) **Noticing the beauty of nature, trees moving, bird chirping and leaves moving, with my senses.**

n) Cooking with awareness of flavors, smells and textures, (cooking with my senses).

o) Having philosophical conversations about the meaning of life with strangers, family, friends or my girlfriend.

4. After you have completed a list of at least fifteen activities, pick your five favorite activities and circle them.

   My favorites are in bold above.

5. Write a brief statement (twenty-five words or so) of your vision of an ideal world. Write this vision in the present tense and in terms of how you want it to be rather than how you want it not to be. Begin your statement this way:
   'An ideal world is one in which…'

   An ideal world is one in which people appreciate each other with kind curiosity for the other's ideas, and ask questions to evolve as a collective awareness unity, where separation and loneliness are non-existent , where kind and courageous acts of love - both intimate and humanitarian - and idea evolution brought about through conversation, drive a feeling of happiness.

6. Now you are going to cut and paste your life purpose together. It's easy and fun. Here you go...
   The purpose of my life is to use my (list the five general characteristics you circled) curiosity, kindness, daring, loving and awareness, *by (list the five specific behaviors)* being affectionate and expressing love to the people I love; exercising awareness of how my thoughts influence my mood and ability to name my thoughts for what they are; using my awareness in conversation and coaching to increase overall awareness in dialogue, helping

others realize how they are thinking and how their words are affecting their thoughts, their interpretations and associations with events, people and relationships; troubleshooting at work to find the right people who can fix the problem and eliminating problems (being a fixer; noticing the beauty of nature, trees moving, bird chirping and leaves moving, with my senses *to bring about a world in which (copy in your ideal world statement)* people appreciate each other with kind curiosity for the others ideas, ask questions in conversation to evolve as a collective awareness unity, where separation and loneliness are rare or non-existent and where kind acts, love – both intimate and humanitarian – and idea evolution brought about through conversation, drive a feeling of happiness.

Summary and tips:
After completing my life purpose statement, I made a couple of small changes. In fact the architect of this exercise recommends tweaking the statement and evolving it regularly to ensure it keeps resonating. I already decided to switch a couple of my favorite five behaviors. This morning I've printed off a copy of the statement and placed it in front of me on my desk at work as both a reminder of my purpose and how I can apply this at work, and as a source of motivation and inspiration.

<u>Conclusion</u>

This project turned out to be more than just twenty-five days of happiness. It's taken me probably thirty days to complete all the exercises but it's helped me transition from a life focus on happiness theory and research to a life focus on the practical application of that theory and research. The exercises I released into the world in *The Happiness Animal* are increasingly embedded in my five happiness muscles' memory. You know what? Now that I've completed the twenty-five exercises, I want to go back and do them again. And practice until they come so naturally that I won't need this book to remind me how to exercise. Twenty-five days of happiness are great, but why not incorporate a little exercise into every day of my life? After finishing my happiness boot camp, I'm not ready to let my five muscles atrophy. I did enjoy some of the exercises more than others, just as I enjoy kayaking more than running on a treadmill, and if I'm honest, I may not repeat some of the exercises again. Instead, I will focus on those I enjoy the most. My commitment now is to stay fit and enjoy both the process and the results, and I recommend you do the same. Happiness, so I've found, is less of an end state, and more of a process. A cliché that holds true: happiness is a journey and not a destination. In the pages that follow, you now have the opportunity to travel through your own twenty-five days of happiness. And I'd love for you to send me a postcard.

Appendix – The Exercises

Chapter 1, Day 1: Exercising sincerity: Be sincere with me dear
Based on exercises for 'Connecting the Range' that appear in the book *Finding your voice* by Barbara Houseman. Barbara is a coach to both Joseph Fiennes and Kenneth Branagh. Reproduced in part with the permission of Nick Hern Books.

Exercise for connecting your voice to your truth, so you speak sincerely. Internally, we may remain as expressive as when we were children, but this inner expression can become 'unplugged' from our outer expression. We may shut down out of fear of being too passionate, too revealing or too emotional. Or we may mask feelings of depression or tiredness or sadness or boredom – exaggerating the pitch movement in our voice so we seem happier or more upbeat than we feel. Either way, our movement around our pitch range fails to truthfully reflect our thoughts and feelings.

We are often not aware of having made a decision to disconnect in this way. So, now, it can be very frustrating, since we don't understand why the life of our internal voice does not show through in the life of our external voice. Another cause of flatness or exaggerated movement in the voice can be lack of trust. One of two behaviors occurs when we lose trust: either we become tentative or we become over-effortful. If we become over-effortful, the voice will tend to be over exaggerated in its pitch movement since we will not trust our thoughts and feelings to be expressed by the natural movement of the voice and will therefore 'help' everything along. A further cause of disconnection can be that we are not connecting with what we are saying or with the person we are saying it to. This can happen both with our own words and with text. We need to see the pictures or images behind our words and, then, we need to *want* the person we are addressing to see the same pictures and images. This is not a question of thinking about what you are saying or trying to *explain* it to your listener. It is about being present with the words and images and with the person you're speaking to. This may sound horrendously complicated but it isn't and when you make this connection you become utterly simple and yet utterly engaging!

You start by exercising your connection with words to fully and authentically color how you say them.

Instructions
1. Sit comfortably, somewhere that is quiet and private.
2. Take a piece of text a small phrase at a time, sometimes you may even take one word at a time. The reason for this is that, if you take more than a few words at once, you will find yourself only connecting with some of the words, usually the 'so called' more important ones. Whereas, if you take a few words at a time you can connect with every word. This does not mean that you will end up stressing every word, but rather that each word will have its own place and color within the whole, which leads to greater variety and greater subtlety.
3. Take the first phrase and repeat it quietly, but not whispered, three times. Just let the words register. Don't try to find different ways to say them, simply let the words sink in.
4. Then, move on to the next phrase and say that three times through, again letting the words sink in and register.
5. Continue in this way, saying each small phrase three times and then moving on to the next.
6. Don't string all the phrases together, just say each one three times and then leave it and move onto the next.
7. There is no need to try and achieve anything in this exercise, just receive the words and let them guide your voice.

Now it's time to share the pictures with the listener. Use the energy of your communication to bring life and authentic color to your speech. The following steps are all about connecting with your listener.

Sincerity is about two connections: firstly connecting with the words, and secondly connecting with your listener. It is these two connections that will bring your full range into play in a truthful and exciting way. You need a partner for the following steps.

8. Sit comfortably opposite your partner
9. Start to speak a piece of text to your partner. Focus on talking rather than acting the text. Put all your attention on your partner and on wanting to communicate with them.

10. As you are talking, your partner listens and honestly questions any part of the text where they don't get the picture. Here is an example of how the exercise might work using some of dialogue from 'Pentecost' by David Edgar.

> YOU: When she came back
> PARTNER: When she what?

11. You then need to answer by repeating the particular bit of text questioned, but you can't raise your voice or emphasize the word (or words) more to get the images across to your partner. You need to really connect with what that word (or words) mean for you, what they conjure up and then share that.

> YOU: came back
> (If your partner feels they have received the picture, you can move on, otherwise they may ask again)
> YOU: at first it looked quite normal
> PARTNER: When did it look quite normal?
> YOU: at first
> (Again, if your partner feels they have received the picture, you can move on, otherwise they may ask again)

> YOU: it looked quite normal
> PARTNER: Looked quite odd?
> YOU: quite normal
> YOU: And as it was the morning
> PARTNER: The evening?
> YOU: the morning
> YOU: it was no surprise to find the door open
> PARTNER: It was a shock?
> PARTNER: it was no surprise
> YOU: to find the door open
> PARTNER: to find the shop door closed?
> YOU: to find the door open

12. Your partner has a big responsibility here to not just question you arbitrarily but to really pick you up when they feel that they haven't been communicated with.

13. Your responsibility is not to take the easy way out and simply raise your voice or emphasize the word more, but rather to really connect with the word and share that.

Chapter 3, Day 2: Exercising harmony in disclosure (connection1.2):
Writing the wrong
Adapted from an exercise that appears in *The Happiness Hypothesis* by
Jonathan Haidt.

Instructions
1. Take a blank piece of paper and write for five minutes about 'the
    most upsetting or traumatic experience of your entire life. If you
    have never experienced trauma, write about something that upset you
    or something you are ashamed of, or, a deep regret. Preferably
    choose an experience you have not talked about with other people in
    much detail, if at all. You don't have to show what you write to
    anyone other than yourself.
2. The next day, continue writing about the experience for another five
    minutes. Don't edit or censor yourself. Don't worry about grammar
    or sentence structure; just keep writing. Write about what happened,
    how you feel about it, and why you feel that way, and in whatever
    order you like.
3. Repeat for several days until you have nothing further to write.

Tip: If you hate to write, talk into a voice recorder on your phone. The
crucial thing is to get your thoughts and feelings out in words without
imposing any order on them – but in such a way that, after a few days, some
order is likely to emerge on its own.

4. If the experience involved another person, ask the other person to
    meet up with you as a favor to you.
5. When you meet up with the other person, notice any bodily
    sensations associated with your anxiety or fear of disclosing what
    you are going to disclose to them. Where do you feel tension? Your
    stomach? Your forehead? Your shoulders? Your hands?
6. Tell the other person that you are doing this to exercise your honesty
    connection, an exercise in disclosure for the benefit of your own
    happiness.
7. When disclosing your story, take your time. Speak slowly and notice
    any bodily sensations you have as and when they come up. If the
    other person reacts to what you say, notice your own body's reaction
    before you react verbally. Tell them how you are feeling throughout

the disclosure. e.g. 'I notice my hands are shaking' or 'I'm feeling tension in my stomach'.

8. If resentments and/or appreciations come up continue this exercise with the exercise of expressing yourself

Chapter 3, Day 3: Exercising integrity (express yourself)

(Based on exercises for Getting Into and Getting Over Anger, in *Radical Honesty*, by Brad Blanton)

1) Close your eyes for a moment, picture a person you don't like, and have an imaginary dialogue with him. Tell him what he did that you resent. Tell him your judgments about him. Then imagine his response and respond back. You may also tell him your appreciations if you have any, or if any show up after your expression of resentment. Pay attention to your body as you engage in this imaginary dialogue. Take a break from reading here and do this step now.

2) Call the person you just had an imaginary conversation with and make an appointment to tell him your resentments in person. Tell the person when you call that you want to meet him to tell him what you are mad about and get over it, and get complete with him. Ask him to meet with you as a favor to you. Persist until he agrees to meet with you.

3) Meet with your enemy. Your goal will be to forgive him not as a favor to him, but for your own selfish benefit.

4) Follow the below guidelines for communication during the meeting. These guidelines are not moral rules to be memorized and obeyed. They are rules of thumb. The purpose of these guidelines is to direct your attention to the process of learning how to express yourself in the moment so that something happens to actual feelings in your body at the level of sensation. Something will happen because of your willingness to pay attention to your experience. These guidelines will make your aware of your moment-to-moment experience of anger or of appreciation. **But beware of your mind.** The rules can be followed and still not work if you are only attending to the rules and not to your experience. The point is to be aware of your

experience while experimenting, not whether you are good at following the rules. Your goal is to be willing and to acknowledge to yourself, and to report with whom you are speaking, each new experience as it emerges, regardless of whether or not it is comfortable. You'll have no more withheld resentments or appreciations, and you'll be able to experience him newly, as he is, in that moment. When you let someone be the way they are, when you let up on your judgments of someone, there is free space in which forgiveness and love can occur. **Here are the rules of thumb for the conversation:**

    I.   Whenever possible, talk face-to-face to the person with whom you are angry. It is impossible to do any of this work over the phone. You need to look at each other in the eye and react to each other moment to moment.

    II.   Start your sentences as often as possible with the words, **'I resent you for...'** or **'I appreciate you for...'** The structure of a sentence that starts with those words ensures that the anger is personal, that there is an 'I' and a 'you'. I resent you has a much stronger and more personal impact than 'I resent the fact that...'

    III.   Speak in the **present tense** (I resent you for ...NOT I resented you for...)

    IV.   **Get specific.** Even though it doesn't always feel this way, you probably resent the person for what he specifically did or said. E.g. Instead of saying: 'I resent you for acting snobbish toward me', to which he can say 'I'm not a snob', say: I resent you for turning your head and not answering me when I said hi to you.'

    V.   Focus as much as you can on what *did* happen instead of what didn't happen.

    VI.   Stay in touch with your experience as you talk. Don't rehearse a speech. Stick to expressing your feelings as they come up during the interaction. What you need to do to tell the truth and have the resentment disappear is this: first, notice the bodily sensations associated with what you have called anger (feeling constricted in your breathing, cowering, feeling tense, frowning) and state your resentment clearly. Start with, 'I resent you for saying....' When you hear yourself say whatever specifically it is you say it may end up sounding ridiculous and unfair. But note this: The unfair blaming is being done out loud. It is in the public domain where it can get cleared up, not in your secretive mind.

VII. **Stay there with the person beyond the time it takes to exchange resentments.** Keep stating your resentments as they come up, and allow the other person to resent you for resenting him, eventually you won't have anything left to resent each other for.

VIII. **After you both have fully expressed your specific resentments, state your appreciation in the same way. Say, 'I appreciate you for...' Not 'I appreciate the fact that....'** Keep checking your body to see how you feel. Are your shoulders tense? Do you feel relaxed? Do you feel like you want to get away from this situation as soon as possible? If the latter is true, there is more that you are withholding. Tell the truth of your experience even if it's: 'I still feel uncomfortable sitting here with you,' or 'I appreciate you for staying here and listening to me'. When you feel warmth in your chest and a smile on your face, express your appreciation in a clear way: 'I appreciate you for the way you look at me right now.' Some more resentments may emerge. If that happens, express those resentments and go on. Eventually you will just be sitting in a room looking at a person. You will see clearer. You be willing to live and let live. You will be grateful to him for having stuck with you through another fight.

IX. **Keep it up.** After an emotional exchange in which people tell the truth, they often retreat into superficiality. Keep up with 'I resent you for...' and 'I appreciate you for ...' as they come up. You will tend to withhold your feelings on later occasions because you have practiced that for years, but you can always clean it up with the person as soon as you realize you are withholding.

Chapter 3, Day 4: call it bullshit.

Exercise for: washing your words
Before you next go to meet up with a friend or a family member, or go into a meeting at work, stop.
First, answer the following questions:

1. What is my intention going into this conversation?

_____

_____

_____

_____

2. Am I operating with a second agenda?
   YES   ~   NO   (circle as appropriate)

3. What is my real motivation for this conversation?

_____

_____

_____

_____

Now, practice doing the following before your actual conversation: Get a chair and sit or stand facing it.

4. Imagine that the other person is sat in the chair. Talk out loud about what you intend to talk about during your conversation with the other person **and start every sentence with either the words 'I notice'**

or **'I imagine'** Restrict the use of 'I notice' to things you can physically notice right now, using your five senses. Be aware of the difference between what you can notice and what you imagine. The rule here is that unless you can actually notice something very specific e.g. you can see a specific sentence written down in front of you then you start your sentences with the words 'I imagine'.

5. Continue your practice conversation with the other person but this time instead of using the words 'I imagine', say 'I bullshit'

6. Meet up with the person. During your actual conversation, practice starting your sentences with either 'I notice' or 'I imagine' and be aware of the difference between the two.

7. Give yourself permission to speak frankly, even if it is abnormal for you to be frank. Focus simply on saying what is so and what you can notice, and the sensations you feel when talking about different topics in the conversation. e.g. 'Now we are talking about KPI8, I notice some tension in my stomach. I imagine it's because I saw…'

Chapter 3, Day 5: Exercising Trust

Exercise for: building trust in yourself and others

Part I – trust yourself (Part I is based on an exercise by psychologist Susanne Babbell)

1. Sit or lie down so that you feel comfortable.

2. Now, how can you make it even more comfortable? Get a blanket, a pillow... whatever will make you feel relaxed and content.

3. Once you are settled, ask yourself: 'How do I know this is comfortable?' This might appear to be a silly question, and perhaps

even confusing. However, it is an important one in increasing your skills of building trust (using your senses, not your mind).

4. Continue to explore what sensation you feel that you recognize as comfort. For example, you might think: 'I do not feel any pain', 'I breathe easily', or 'I feel relaxed'.

5. You might be anticipating that this feeling won't last, which is true. We can't control or grasp onto this pleasurable feeling. It's only important that you are in the present moment right now, not drifting into thoughts of the future or the past. Thinking of the future can create anxiety; thinking of the past can create depression.

6. Remain aware of any sounds, the temperature, the light, and your physical sensations. Can you let yourself simply enjoy the moment?

7. You can practice this exercise for as long as you prefer and as time allows you. Just keep checking in with your level of comfort. What feelings indicate that you are comfortable? With time, you will start to trust your feelings (your senses) again.

Part II – Trust that you can trust others

8. At the next opportunity, ask a family member or a colleague if they can get you (or make you) the hot drink of your choice. And trust that they can do it for you.

9. Meet with a friend and confide in them with a secret. Even if there is a risk they could tell someone else, trust that they won't. Tell them

you trust that they won't tell anyone and that you are putting your trust in them by telling them this.

10. Lend a favorite possession to a friend and trust that they will look after it and give it back to you, e.g. your favorite book, DVD, or an appliance. You could lend them your coffee machine or crêpe maker while you are on holiday.

11. Practice these trusting body language exercises: **a) eye contact** with a colleague, friend, or loved one: ask the other person to stand facing you and to stare into your eyes while you stare back for one minute; **b) eye contact with touch** – repeat step a) but this time hold hands as well; **c) proximity** – this time stand opposite the other person a comfortable distance apart, and then ask the other person to move a little closer and notice how what you feel changes as they move closer. Then increase the distance and notice how it changes how you feel.

Chapter 4, Day 6: 4 smiles, 4 hugs and a cup of tea: exercising warmth (connection2.1)

Exercise for when you are feeling lonely, cold, or isolated. This is an exercise that warms up your daily routine.

Instructions
Hugs: Offer to give someone you know (or someone you don't know but would be comfortable hugging) a hug: 1) in the morning 2) at lunch 3) in the afternoon 4) in the evening. Ask as many different people as you feel comfortable hugging.
Smiles: On the way to work (in the car, while walking, on the bus) smile at least one person. Do the same on your lunch break, and again on the way home from work.
Cup of tea: In the office, or at home: If someone seems stressed, upset or just tired, tell them you are making a cup of tea for yourself and them and ask what kind of tea they drink. Go get it and bring it back to them. Alternatively if you happen to see someone crying out on the street, at the bus stop or train station (and you feel comfortable talking to them), approach them and ask them what the matter is. Offer them a hug and a 'let's get you a cup of tea'. Buy them a cup, and then say goodbye with a smile.

Chapter 4, Day 7: Exercising respect: hear me now

Exercise for any face-to-face conversation. This is an exercise in active listening and giving your full attention. It is an exercise in not disagreeing out loud if your first reaction is to disagree with what's being said. It is an exercise in respecting that this is simply what the other person is saying. It is impossible to disagree that someone is saying the words they are saying to you. If, during this exercise you find yourself tempted to disagree with the person you are listening to, simply repeat back what the other says: if your child says, 'I don't want to go to school today', you say to your child, 'you don't want to go to school today' (instead of the common response: 'of course you do') . In Gretchen Rubin's *The Happiness Project*, she describes this as 'Acknowledge the reality of people's feelings'. Gretchen's strategies for acknowledging the reality of people's feelings are: 1) write down what the other person says to you; 2) don't feel as if you have to say anything; 3) don't say 'no' or 'stop'; 4) admit that tasks that the other person says they are finding it hard to do, are difficult (by replying to them with comments like 'yes it is not easy to do that'). Try and make use of these four strategies in the following exercise:

Instructions
1. Before you start listening, imagine your head full of the thoughts you have right now.
2. Imagine that you are starting to pull the huge lever for your thoughts to the off position. As you get closer to off, it will spring to that position with force on its own. Imagine the noise of the power springing to off.
3. Now you have switched off, you are ready to receive power from the other person. Now you are ready to begin to notice things that are not your own thoughts or ideas.
    TIP: If you find thoughts creeping back in – acknowledge them and accept them. To bring your presence back, notice the feeling of your breath going in and out of your body. Relax your shoulders. This will be enough to bring you into being present with the person who is speaking. Don't make an effort to breath. Just notice three of your breaths in and out, the pauses in between, and the feeling as the air rushes inside.
4. Notice which parts of the speaker's body are moving as you listen to them. Notice their hands, their ears, their jaw, their cheeks, their eyebrows. Pay attention to all their movements and acknowledge

them to yourself. Watch for eye movements as the other person talks to you.

5. Paraphrase back what the other person has just said to you every time they pause.

Regularly ask a question that takes the form of repeating back what the person just said to you that shows your understanding. Try opening your question with 'So you ....' and ending your question with a smile and a 'Is that right?'

Chapter 4, Day 8: Exercising recognition and appreciation - I appreciate you

Exercise for: Anytime you are around other people (strangers, family or friends)

1. Identify an individual. It could be someone you are talking with, or a complete stranger.
2. List 3 body movements you notice in the individual. **Tip: look at their hands, feet, eyebrows, jaw, shoulders, neck, mouth.**

1)_____

_____

2)_____

_____

3)

_____

3. List one of the body movements or positions you also notice as similar in yourself. If you can't notice something similar, write how you differ in one of the body movements.

_____

4. List one description – physical, verbal, or behavioral of the individual that you appreciate them for e.g. (their eyes, smile, hand position, posture)
   I appreciate their

5. Make eye contact with the person, smile and tell them what you appreciate them for. Start your sentence with 'I appreciate your_____' or 'I appreciate you for _____. **Note:** If you feel too awkward to give verbal appreciation to a stranger, simply acknowledge the other person with a smile or a nod when you make eye contact with them.

Chapter 4, Day 9: A tissue! Exercising kindness with the ABC of Gratitude

Exercise for on a train, on the beach, in the café, in the supermarket, in the queue, or at home. You will need a pack of tissues for this exercise.

Instructions:
1. Watch for anyone who could use a tissue (someone spilling something on themselves, sniffing their runny nose, sneezing, suffering from hay fever, or crying).
2. Take your pack of tissues out so it is clearly visible in your hand.
3. Notice any tension areas in your body and relax those areas. Imagine your shoulder blades dropping gently down your back, and that all your joints are loose. Smile.
4. Approach the person with a smile, make eye contact, and ask them 'would you like a tissue?' Offer the pack of tissues towards them.
5. If they take the tissue and thank you, notice how you feel. If they don't, start again from step 1.

Note: If you don't have any tissues with you, you can exercise by simply anticipating and then offering assistance e.g. if you are in a café and someone with a laptop is looking around the café, you can tell them what the wifi code is. Or if you see someone coming to your building with a lot of bags or boxes, offer to help them carry their things, or if you anticipate that they will need help getting in, hold the doors open for them. If you are in the supermarket and someone seems fidgety or anxious in the queue, perhaps looking at their watch, offer to let them go ahead of you. It doesn't matter what you exercise with, the key is how you exercise: anticipate and then offer help.

Chapter 4, Day 10: musical chairs

Exercise for empathy: You can do this exercise to empathize with anyone, and it works well if you have had a difficulty with someone important in your life, such as an argument with your significant other, or parents.

Instructions
1. Arrange two chairs facing each other.
2. Sit in one chair. This is your chair. Imagine the other person you want to exercise empathy with is sat opposite you.
3. What do you want to say to the other person you want to empathize with? Say it to them now, as if they were there. Stay honest, and make your comments as specific as possible. (If you have anger or resentment you want to express, use the language from the exercise in connection 1.3).
4. Focus your attention on the other chair imagining the other person is sat there right now as you talk to them. You may feel silly at first, but feeling silly is your trigger to drop your protective ego. If you feel silly, it is because you are not dropping your guard enough to empathize yet. Talk like no one's watching (in this case no one is watching!).
5. Now, get up and sit in the other chair. Imagine you are the other person and respond back to the other chair. Focus your attention as you talk on the other chair imagining that you (as seen through the eyes of the other person) are sitting there.
6. Repeat steps 3 & 4 until you have said everything you'd like to say to the other person, and have responded back as the other person from the other chair. Every time you respond in step 5, you are empathizing with the other person, imagining what they would be thinking and feeling and what they would say to you.

When I do this exercise I often feel an emotional wave coming over me when I respond as the other. It's the warmth of empathy of understanding another person. This exercise is also great for exercising tolerance of others and gives your Five connections' tolerance, kindness and honesty connections a workout all at the same time.

Additional steps for exercising compassion:
Continue with the use of the two chairs placed opposite each other.

1. Sit in 'your' chair and imagine the suffering of anyone you know. If the person is different to the person you exercised empathy with, complete the empathy steps (above) for the new person first.

2. Now, get up and sit in the other chair. Imagine that you are the one suffering.

3. Reflect on how much you would like your suffering to end.

4. Now imagine the person in the chair opposite would like your suffering to end. What would you like for that person to do to end your suffering?

5. Switch chairs. You are you again. Focus on the chair opposite, imagining the other (suffering) person sat there. Imagine what you would like to do for the other person's suffering to end. Imagine doing something to help ease their suffering. If you want to, talk to the other chair as you did in the empathy steps. If you feel even a little that you'd want their suffering to end, reflect on that feeling. With exercise and experiencing the warmth of this feeling, your kindness connection, and your Five connections will flourish.

Once you get good at step 5, practice doing something small each day to help end the suffering of others, by imagining what it's like living in their body, and what they would want someone else to do to help. It could be as simple as picking up some groceries, getting their lunch, or giving them a lift home from work.

Chapter 5, Day 11: Exercising tolerance with fear - Life through a lens. From telephoto to wide angle

Exercise for when you are trigger-happy with your zoom button, and would benefit from switching to a wide angle lens. Instead of zooming in on one fear, you can see what's in the bigger picture: your lifescape. Human beings have a tendency to be trigger-happy and over-zoom, so this exercise helps you to zoom out your magnification back to the natural 1x of your senses.

Instructions:
2. Write down a current fear or anxiety in the middle of a blank sheet of paper.
3. Using a pencil, draw one circle at a time around your fear.
4. Notice how your circles are forced to get bigger each time you draw another circle around the previous one. This is exactly what happens in your mind: The more attention, questions, thoughts, associations, and links you give a problem, the more space the problem takes up in your mind, the more the problem dominates your being.
5. Erase the circles one by one starting with the largest circle, until you are left only with the word that's been causing your fear.
6. Using the free space on the paper that was previously taken up by your unnecessary circles, write down the name of someone whose company you value.
7. Write down the name of something you would enjoy doing for that person.
8. Write down when you can do it.
9. Using more of the newly freed-up space, write down the name of an interest you enjoy and feel drawn to finding out more about.
10. Look back at the fear that you have written down. What was more detrimental to you, the fear or your circles of zoom around the fear?
11. Were the circles of zoom unnecessary?
12. Were the circles not leaving much space for the good things in your life?
13. Laugh at yourself. Laugh at yourself for drawing unnecessary circles around something that just is.
14. Laugh. No seriously, laugh. Laughter has been clinically proven to reduce the stress hormones cortisol and adrenaline, hormones linked to medical problems such as adrenal fatigue, high blood pressure, and depression. Laughter relaxes blood pressure and increases immune system activity by increasing the release of interferon.

Still suffering with thoughts of fear and anxiety? Reality test your fear and anxiety:
1. What is the worst that can happen?

_____

_____

2. How likely is it, that the worst will happen, based on my experience on a scale of one to ten, with ten being most likely?

1   2   3   4   5   6   7   8   9   10

3. What can I do to reduce the likelihood of this happening?

_____

_____

_____

4. Can I survive the worst and live with it if it does happen?

Yes I can survive this   No I won't survive

5. If you said no to question four, have you ever not survived anything in the past?

Yes   No

6. If you said no to question five, what makes you think you won't survive something this time?

_____

_____

_____

7. Laugh at yourself. Laugh at yourself for giving so much attention to one piece of your life that represents infinitely less than a dot in the universe. Good, now you're not feeling as anxious, it's a great time to talk about one of the most frequent sources of human anxiety and fear: Pain.

Chapter 5, Day 12: Exercising tolerance with pain

Exercise for when you are finding it hard to think about anything other than how much pain you are feeling.

Deep Breathing: Breathing is the bedrock of yoga. Yoga has been around for three thousand years. And it's never been more popular than today. But I also know that amongst my readers there are likely to be more than just a handful of yoga skeptics, dismissing yoga as wishy washy or hokus pokus, aka non-scientific bullshit. But yoga can be analyzed scientifically, more specifically in terms of its biological benefits. Google it. It has been around for three millennia so you'd kind of expect some criticism, but there is also scientific validation. So back to my point: you don't have to believe in yoga to benefit from this book, but this is the one exercise in the book that uses principles from yoga to take your attention and focus away from pain. If you are not in pain, you can use discomfort of any kind, or bookmark this exercise as a tool you can use like a first aid kit.

Pre-exercise: If I didn't feel pain, what feeling would I be left with right now? Write your answer below:

_____

_____

_____

_____

Exercise Instructions (adapted from: *The Science of Breath*)

8. Sit upright, in an easy posture, being sure to hold the chest, neck and head in a straight a line as possible, with shoulders slightly back and

hands resting easily on the lap. In this position the weight of the body is largely supported by the ribs and the position may be easily maintained. Yoga instructors have found that you cannot get the best effect of rhythmic breathing with the chest drawn in and the abdomen protruding.

9. Breathing through the nostrils (it is important to keep your nostrils clear all the time and breath through them as much of the time as possible), inhale steadily, first filling the lower part of the lungs, pushing out the lower ribs, breast bone and chest. Then fill the highest portion of the lungs, protruding the upper chest, thus lifting up the chest, including the upper six or seven pairs of ribs. In the final movement, the lower part of the abdomen will be slightly drawn in, which movement gives the lungs a support and also helps to fill the highest part of the lungs. The inhalation is continuous, the entire chest cavity from the lowered diaphragm to the highest point of the chest in the region of the collar bone, being expanded with a uniform movement. Avoid a jerky series of inhalations, and strive to attain a steady, continuous action. Practice will soon overcome the tendency to divide the inhalation into three movements, and will result in a uniform continuous breath. You will be able to complete the inhalation in a couple of seconds after a little practice.

10. Retain the breath for a few seconds.

11. Exhale quite slowly, holding the chest in a firm position, and drawing the abdomen in a little and lifting it upward slowly as the air leaves the lungs. When the air is entirely exhaled, relax the chest and abdomen. A little practice will make this part of the exercise easy, and the movement once acquired will later be performed almost automatically.

12. Steps 1-4 are called a 'Complete Breath' in Yoga. Now we make it rhythmical. Repeat step 2 again, but this time as you inhale count six beats of your pulse. Then retain the breath for three beats of your pulse.

13. Exhale slowly through the nostrils over a period of six beats of your pulse.

14. Count three pulse beats between breaths.

15. Repeat steps 5-7 a number of times, but avoid tiring yourself out.

16. Once you have established a rhythm, feel an intention inside you (if you believe in will power, this is the time to use it – if you don't, just be aware of yourself having an intention to follow the next instruction. Use your will power or intention to carry this thought:

Each inhalation is drawing an increased supply of energy from not just the oxygen, but all the other stuff you are breathing in. It is a fact of physics, that there is energy in the air you breath because atoms in the air you breath are vibrating. Vibrations are energy. This is literally, not metaphorically, energy of the universe (universal energy), which is taken up by your nervous system.

17. On the exhalation, will the thought, or be aware of your intention, to send the universal energy you have inhaled to the painful part of your body, to re-establish the circulation and nerve current.
18. Inhale more of the universal energy for the purpose of driving out the painful condition, then exhale, holding the thought that you are driving out the pain.
19. Alternate between the two mental commands with each exhalation: on the first exhalation, re-establish the circulation and nerve current; on the next exhalation, drive out the pain.
20. Repeat step 12 for seven breaths.
21. On the next inhalation, retain the air for a few seconds. Then pucker up your lips as if you were going to whistle (but do not puff out the cheeks), then exhale a little air through the opening with short, sharp force. Stop exhaling for a moment, retaining the air, and then exhale a little more air. Repeat this stop-start exhalation until the air is completely exhaled. Remember to use considerable vigor, exhaling through the puckered opening of the lips. Yoga instructors call this step the cleansing breath.
22. Rest for a minute.
23. Repeat steps 11 and 12 and this time continue until pain relief comes, which will be before long. Many pains will be relieved before seven breaths are finished. If the hand is placed over the painful part, you may get quicker results. Send the current of universal energy you have inhaled down the arm and into the painful part through your hand.

Chapter 5, Day 13: Exercising tolerance of others: all in the same boat

Exercise for tolerating other people

Instructions
Do this exercise if your first reaction is one of disdain or dismissal towards anyone. For example it could be a reaction in your self of disgust towards a shaved haircut, a beard, a tattoo, a loud voice or colored hair.

1. Look at the person. Notice your reaction. Notice the physical sensations in your body of that reaction and stay with those sensations for 30 seconds (or until they disappear).

2. With your attention geared to the other person, tell yourself the following in this order (from 'Just Like Me' by Harry Palmer):

    a. 'Just like me, this person is seeking happiness in his/her life.'
    b. 'Just like me, this person is trying to avoid suffering in his/her life.'
    c. 'Just like me, this person has known sadness, loneliness and despair.'
    d. 'Just like me, this person is seeking to fill his/her needs.'
    e. 'Just like me, this person is learning about life.'

3. Look back at the person. Notice any movements they make. Start at their feet and check each body part. Notice any movements in different parts of their body. What are they doing with their hands? Their fingers? Their shoulders? What internal feelings do you think those bodily movements relate to? Do you notice any movements in them that you recognize in yourself?

Notice your own body. How have the sensations changed from your first reaction (in step 1).

Chapter 5, Day 14: Exercising patience - a plant, a jug, five mugs and a teaspoon

Patience can't be acquired overnight. It is just like building up a connection. Every day you need to work on it

Eknath Easwaran

Oddly enough, the exercises for tolerance of pain and tolerance of fear also work for exercising patience at the time you are feeling impatient. Practice using those exercises as tools whenever you are already feeling the impatience. To use an asthma analogy, the exercises for tolerance of pain and fear are the Vent(olin) relievers for feelings of pain, fear and impatience. The following is more a preventative exercise for impatience, the brown steroid inhaler or Becotide, that works best when you are not already feeling impatient but will prepare you and increase your resilience to future impatience triggers. This exercise is based on a Tibetan Buddhist meditation ritual. You can try the original ritual but you will need to find five hundred tiny bottles first. Given I don't know anyone who keeps five hundred empty bottles around their house, I have adapted this exercise.

You will need: a large plant, a jug, five mugs and a teaspoon. If you don't have a plant to water, use the nearest tree or lawn.

Instructions:
1) Fill five mugs to the brim with water.
2) Carry the full mugs one at a time over to where the plant is and put them down slowly. Imagine you are doing it as calmly as you possibly can, making sure you are breathing easily through your nose, while you focus on not spilling any water.
3) Pick up the teaspoon and the first of the five mugs.
4) Take one teaspoon of water at a time out of the mug and feed it to the plant, lawn or tree. Focus entirely on the spoon and the water (and not spilling the water). Continue spooning until the mug is empty.
5) Put down the empty mug and pick up the next mug and repeat step 4.
6) Repeat step 4 and 5 until all mugs are empty.

Chapter 5, Day 15: Exercising tolerance of self - Curiosity and self-forgiveness

Exercise for challenging limiting beliefs about you, and for forgiving you.

Instructions

Part I – Noticing the difference between what you can notice and what you imagine about yourself

1. Write down five sentences that begin with the words **'I notice...'** Whatever you notice must be something you can physically notice **about yourself** with your senses (vision, hearing, taste, smell or touch, right now in this present moment). You can't notice

something that happened in the past or in the future. Write these sentences down below.

e.g. I notice an itch on my inner thigh

1.

___

2.

___

3.

___

4.

___

5.

___

2. Now write down five sentences starting with the words 'I imagine'. Each sentence is about one thing you **imagine about yourself**.

e.g. I imagine I am a bad in bed with my girlfriend; I imagine I am a loser; I imagine I won't get the job; I imagine I am a failure.

1.

___

2.

___

3.

___

4.

_____

_____

5.

_____

_____

3. How many of the negative things or limiting beliefs you have written about yourself are things you imagine vs. things you can actually notice in this moment?
   _____things I notice about myself, _____ I imagine about myself are negative.

Part II - Optional additional exercise for self forgiveness

Exercise for when you can't forgive yourself for something. Adapted from an exercise by Jonathan Haidt in *The Happiness Hypothesis.*

It's important to go into this exercise with an awareness that you don't have to show what you write to anyone, so there is no need to be afraid of what you are writing. Brené Brown says that shame needs three things to grow exponentially: Secrecy, silence, and judgment. If you put these three ingredients into a Petri dish, they will grow shame. This is an exercise to break your secrecy, silence and judgment, which are making it impossible for you to forgive yourself. If you hate to write, talk into an audio recording device. The crucial thing is to get your thoughts and feelings out in words without imposing any order on them, but in such a way that after a few days some order is likely to emerge on its own.

Instructions
1. Take a blank piece of paper and write the words: 'I can't forgive myself for....' at the top of one of the pages.
2. Choose one thing you are struggling to forgive yourself for. It could be something minor in the context of your whole life or it could be something you are ashamed of that happened today, or it could be a

deep regret from your past. Preferably choose an experience you have not talked about with other people.

3. Finish the sentence 'I can't forgive myself for....' by adding a brief summary of what you can't forgive yourself for.

4. Take up to five minutes to write, freely, without pausing to edit what you write, about what reasons may have led to you doing the thing you can't forgive yourself for. Try and remember what you had been doing prior to the thing you are trying to forgive yourself for. What was going on in your life around that time? Try and identify at least one reason why you would have done what you did.

5. Now write freely about the reasons you have for not forgiving yourself. What is preventing you from forgiving yourself now?

6. Write about what good you can derive from what you did, about any feelings you have about what you did, and write in any order as the thoughts come to you.

7. Repeat steps 4-6 of writing continuously for up to five minutes a day for several days. Don't edit or censor yourself. Don't worry about grammar or sentence structure; just keep writing. Write about what happened, how you feel about it, and why you feel that way, and in whatever order you like.

8. Before you conclude your last day of writing (you will know it's your last day when you have nothing more to write about it) be sure you have done your best to answer these two questions: Why did this happen? What good might I derive from it?

9. If you still feel guilty, check to see if you still are imagining anger from the person you offended. Check to see if this anger you imagine they have towards you, is actually the anger you feel towards them. Often the source of guilt is anger you feel but have not expressed towards someone else. Brad Blanton explains that often mistakes are made out of anger and that people who are perennial screw ups are usually angry people.

10. Now think about a friend (imaginary or real) who is unconditionally loving, accepting, kind and compassionate. Imagine that this friend can see all your strengths and all your weaknesses, including the details of yourself you have just been writing about. Reflect upon what this friend feels towards you, and how you are loved and accepted exactly as you are, with all your very human imperfections. This friend recognizes the limits of human nature, and is kind and forgiving towards you. In his or her great wisdom this friend understands your life history and the millions of things that have

happened in your life to create you as you are in this moment. Your particular inadequacy is connected to so many things you didn't necessarily choose: your genes, your family history, life circumstances – things that were outside of your control.

11. Write a letter to yourself from the perspective of this friend – focusing on the perceived inadequacy you tend to judge yourself for. If it helps, do this using the model of the musical chairs exercise you used for empathy, and actually get up and switch chairs when you go to write the letter. What would this friend say to you about your "flaw" from the perspective of unlimited compassion? How would this friend convey the deep compassion he or she feels for you, for the pain you feel when you judge yourself so harshly? What would this friend write in order to remind you that you are only human, that all people have both strengths and weaknesses?

12. Add to the letter any suggestions for possible changes, and as you write from the perspective of this friend, be aware of how these suggestions would embody feelings of unconditional understanding and compassion. Try to infuse the letter with a strong sense of acceptance, kindness, caring, and desire of your friend for your health and happiness.

13. After writing the letter, put it down and leave it alone for a few hours or days. Then come back and read it again, really letting the words sink in. Feel the compassion as it pours into you, soothing and comforting you like a hot drink on a cold day. Love, connection and acceptance are your birthright. To claim them you need only look within yourself.

14. Finally, ask yourself: Am I more valuable to others as a vulnerable human being, who is still willing to step into the arena, who is willing to dare to do better but who admits to making mistakes, or as someone who hides secrets and poisons themselves with their own self-judgment and shame?

15. Share your story. People like to know they are not alone in not being perfect. Vulnerability is the strength of a human being who knows they are not perfect but dares greatly nonetheless. Showing vulnerability to the world, as Brené Brown says, is the most accurate measure of courage.

Chapter 6, Day 16: Exercising awareness with FAD (Food, Alcohol and Drugs - the tempting way to self-control

Exercise for when you feel compelled to consume something that you know isn't healthy for your body, nor for your happiness, nor your authenticity.

Instructions
Pause before acting. Take a Being Time Out and do the following.

3. Notice the sensations in your body associated with your feelings and thoughts compelling you to consume. What feelings (e.g. tension in my forehead) are you feeling in different parts of your body?

    _____

    _____

    _____

    _____

1. What do you feel is your inadequacy? Try and define your source of feelings of inadequacy as specifically as possible. Are they sourced in fear of something? What are your thoughts associated with this fear?

    _____

    _____

    _____

    _____

3. How do you feel consuming will help with this inadequacy?

    _____

    _____

    _____

4. Before you consume, ask yourself the following four questions:

    A. Will it bring me power of the genuine [internally authentic] sort?

    B. Will it increase my level of enlightenment?

    C. Will it make me more whole?

    D. Will it make me more loving?

10. Now notice with your senses what your body wants. If your connections feel tired, it could be sleep. If your throat is dry, it could be water. If you have pressure in your bladder or your bowels, maybe you want to go to the toilet. Write it down here:

11. Is what you wrote down in step 6 different to what your mind wants you to consume? The secret to releasing yourself from excess is to start living from what you notice you want rather than what your mind says you should want.

12. Now go back and repeat step 2. Focus on the physical sensations you are having that your mind is associating with the compulsion to consume. Rate your level of pain or discomfort of not giving into the compulsion to consume on a level of 1-10 with 10 being intolerable agony and preferring to die.

13. Reality test your pain/discomfort. Can you live with it? Can you survive it?

14. Allow yourself to fully experience and notice those sensations now. The more you allow yourself to experience them, the more they will have been experienced fully and therefore disappear of their own accord. The alternative, which is resisting those sensations, allows those sensations to persist. The only way to ease them is to allow yourself to experience each physical sensation individually and to stop resisting its perceived unpleasantness. Your mind is a drama queen. The sensations are never as bad as you think they are. It helps if you notice when each sensation appears in your body and if you describe each sensation individually. Describe each sensation below now and then focus your attention on each in turn. Allow yourself to fully experience (and feel) each sensation.

_____

_____

_____

_____

_____

Chapter 6, Day 17: PART I exercising awareness with doing - the conscious veto

Exercise for clearing your mind of distraction and moderating what gets into your to-do list. The more things you feel you should and shouldn't do, the further and further behind your expectations of yourself you fall, the more you shit on yourself, and the more demoralized you feel.

Instructions
1. Look at your to do list if you have one (if not skip to step 3). Mark only those items that are an absolute necessity to you and your family staying alive with an 'N' for necessity. Mark the things you

think you should do with an 'S' for SHIT. One of the Golden rules of the Five connections is that when you should on yourself, you shit on yourself. Shitting on yourself is fairly demoralizing. Mark those things you genuinely want to do with a 'W' for want.

2. Look at your list again. Choose some of the 'S' items to veto and cross them off your list. What remains is more of what you want or need to do.

3. Practice this for the next week: every time you have a thought to do something, ask yourself if it is something you want or need to do. If it isn't, veto it. If you can notice the origin of the thought –what previous thoughts caused you to have that thought? Be aware that you are noticing yourself having the thought to do whatever it is, and you are consciously choosing to veto it.

PART II (from a Harvard Health Report on Positive Psychology)

To keep the burden of choice from robbing you of pleasure, go on a choice diet. For choices of no great consequence, limit the amount of time or number of options you'll consider. Cut off your opportunities for second guessing: stop looking at car or employment ads after you've made a commitment; go ahead and wrap or mail that gift; wear and launder your new pants so they can't be returned. When critical medical or financial choices need to be made, that's the time to put your maximizer tendencies to work. But for the many small choices you make each day, try to narrow your choices quickly and make your decisions confidently.

Chapter 6, Day 18: Exercising tolerance of others - all in the same boat

Exercise for tolerating other people

Instructions
Do this exercise if your first reaction is one of disdain or dismissal towards anyone. For example it could be a reaction in your self of disgust towards a shaved haircut, a beard, a tattoo, a loud voice or colored hair.

1. Look at the person. Notice your reaction. Notice the physical sensations in your body of that reaction and stay with those sensations for 30 seconds (or until they disappear).

2. With your attention geared to the other person, tell yourself the following in this order (from 'Just Like Me' by Harry Palmer):

    a. 'Just like me, this person is seeking happiness in his/her life.'
    b. 'Just like me, this person is trying to avoid suffering in his/her life.'
    c. 'Just like me, this person has known sadness, loneliness and despair.'
    d. 'Just like me, this person is seeking to fill his/her needs.'
    e. 'Just like me, this person is learning about life.'

3. Look back at the person. Notice any movements they make. Start at their feet and check each body part. Notice any movements in different parts of their body. What are they doing with their hands? Their fingers? Their shoulders? What internal feelings do you think those bodily movements relate to? Do you notice any movements in them that you recognize in yourself?

4. Notice your own body. How have the sensations changed from your first reaction (in step 1).

Chapter 6, Day 19: Exercising patience - a plant, a jug, five mugs and a teaspoon

Patience can't be acquired overnight. It is just like building up a connection. Every day you need to work on it

Eknath Easwaran

Oddly enough, the exercises for tolerance of pain and tolerance of fear also work for exercising patience at the time you are feeling impatient. Practice using those exercises as tools whenever you are already feeling the impatience. To use an asthma analogy, the exercises for tolerance of pain and fear are the Vent(olin) relievers for feelings of pain, fear and impatience. The following is more a preventative exercise for impatience, the brown steroid inhaler or Becotide, that works best when you are not already feeling impatient but will prepare you and increase your resilience to future impatience triggers. This exercise is based on a Tibetan Buddhist meditation ritual. You can try the original ritual but you will need to find five hundred tiny bottles first. Given I don't know anyone who keeps five hundred empty bottles around their house, I have adapted this exercise.

You will need: a large plant, a jug, five mugs and a teaspoon. If you don't have a plant to water, use the nearest tree or lawn.

Instructions:
1) Fill five mugs to the brim with water.
2) Carry the full mugs one at a time over to where the plant is and put them down slowly. Imagine you are doing it as calmly as you possibly can, making sure you are breathing easily through your nose, while you focus on not spilling any water.
3) Pick up the teaspoon and the first of the five mugs.
4) Take one teaspoon of water at a time out of the mug and feed it to the plant, lawn or tree. Focus entirely on the spoon and the water (and not spilling the water). Continue spooning until the mug is empty.
5) Put down the empty mug and pick up the next mug and repeat step 4.
6) Repeat step 4 and 5 until all mugs are empty.

Chapter 6, Day 20: Exercising tolerance of self - Curiosity and self-forgiveness

Exercise for challenging limiting beliefs about you, and for forgiving you.

Instructions

Part I – Noticing the difference between what you can notice and what you imagine about yourself

4. Write down five sentences that begin with the words '**I notice...**' Whatever you notice must be something you can physically notice **about yourself** with your senses (vision, hearing, taste, smell or touch, right now in this present moment). You can't notice something that happened in the past or in the future. Write these sentences down below.

   e.g. I notice an itch on my inner thigh
   1.

2.

3.

4.

5.

5. Now write down five sentences starting with the words 'I imagine'.
    Each sentence is about one thing you **imagine about yourself**.
    e.g. I imagine I am a bad in bed with my girlfriend; I
    imagine I am a loser; I imagine I won't get the job; I
    imagine I am a failure.

1.

2.

3.

4.

5. _____

_____

_____

6. How many of the negative things or limiting beliefs you have written about yourself are things you imagine vs. things you can actually notice in this moment?

_____things I notice about myself, _____ I imagine about myself are negative.

Part II - Optional additional exercise for self forgiveness

Exercise for when you can't forgive yourself for something. Adapted from an exercise by Jonathan Haidt in *The Happiness Hypothesis.*

It's important to go into this exercise with an awareness that you don't have to show what you write to anyone, so there is no need to be afraid of what you are writing. Brené Brown says that shame needs three things to grow exponentially: Secrecy, silence, and judgment. If you put these three ingredients into a Petri dish, they will grow shame. This is an exercise to break your secrecy, silence and judgment, which are making it impossible for you to forgive yourself. If you hate to write, talk into an audio recording device. The crucial thing is to get your thoughts and feelings out in words without imposing any order on them, but in such a way that after a few days some order is likely to emerge on its own.

Instructions

16. Take a blank piece of paper and write the words: 'I can't forgive myself for....' at the top of one of the pages.
17. Choose one thing you are struggling to forgive yourself for. It could be something minor in the context of your whole life or it could be something you are ashamed of that happened today, or it could be a deep regret from your past. Preferably choose an experience you have not talked about with other people.
18. Finish the sentence 'I can't forgive myself for....' by adding a brief summary of what you can't forgive yourself for.

19. Take up to five minutes to write, freely, without pausing to edit what you write, about what reasons may have led to you doing the thing you can't forgive yourself for. Try and remember what you had been doing prior to the thing you are trying to forgive yourself for. What was going on in your life around that time? Try and identify at least one reason why you would have done what you did.

20. Now write freely about the reasons you have for not forgiving yourself. What is preventing you from forgiving yourself now?

21. Write about what good you can derive from what you did, about any feelings you have about what you did, and write in any order as the thoughts come to you.

22. Repeat steps 4-6 of writing continuously for up to five minutes a day for several days. Don't edit or censor yourself. Don't worry about grammar or sentence structure; just keep writing. Write about what happened, how you feel about it, and why you feel that way, and in whatever order you like.

23. Before you conclude your last day of writing (you will know it's your last day when you have nothing more to write about it) be sure you have done your best to answer these two questions: Why did this happen? What good might I derive from it?

24. If you still feel guilty, check to see if you still are imagining anger from the person you offended. Check to see if this anger you imagine they have towards you, is actually the anger you feel towards them. Often the source of guilt is anger you feel but have not expressed towards someone else. Brad Blanton explains that often mistakes are made out of anger and that people who are perennial screw ups are usually angry people.

25. Now think about a friend (imaginary or real) who is unconditionally loving, accepting, kind and compassionate. Imagine that this friend can see all your strengths and all your weaknesses, including the details of yourself you have just been writing about. Reflect upon what this friend feels towards you, and how you are loved and accepted exactly as you are, with all your very human imperfections. This friend recognizes the limits of human nature, and is kind and forgiving towards you. In his or her great wisdom this friend understands your life history and the millions of things that have happened in your life to create you as you are in this moment. Your particular inadequacy is connected to so many things you didn't necessarily choose: your genes, your family history, life circumstances – things that were outside of your control.

26. Write a letter to yourself from the perspective of this friend – focusing on the perceived inadequacy you tend to judge yourself for. If it helps, do this using the model of the musical chairs exercise you used for empathy, and actually get up and switch chairs when you go to write the letter. What would this friend say to you about your "flaw" from the perspective of unlimited compassion? How would this friend convey the deep compassion he or she feels for you, for the pain you feel when you judge yourself so harshly? What would this friend write in order to remind you that you are only human, that all people have both strengths and weaknesses?

27. Add to the letter any suggestions for possible changes, and as you write from the perspective of this friend, be aware of how these suggestions would embody feelings of unconditional understanding and compassion. Try to infuse the letter with a strong sense of acceptance, kindness, caring, and desire of your friend for your health and happiness.

28. After writing the letter, put it down and leave it alone for a few hours or days. Then come back and read it again, really letting the words sink in. Feel the compassion as it pours into you, soothing and comforting you like a hot drink on a cold day. Love, connection and acceptance are your birthright. To claim them you need only look within yourself.

29. Finally, ask yourself: Am I more valuable to others as a vulnerable human being, who is still willing to step into the arena, who is willing to dare to do better but who admits to making mistakes, or as someone who hides secrets and poisons themselves with their own self-judgment and shame?

30. Share your story. People like to know they are not alone in not being perfect. Vulnerability is the strength of a human being who knows they are not perfect but dares greatly nonetheless. Showing vulnerability to the world, as Brené Brown says, is the most accurate measure of courage.

Chapter 7, Day 21: Exercising awareness with FAD (Food, Alcohol and Drugs - the tempting way to self-control

Exercise for when you feel compelled to consume something that you know isn't healthy for your body, nor for your happiness, nor your authenticity.

Instructions

Pause before acting. Take a Being Time Out and do the following.

4. Notice the sensations in your body associated with your feelings and thoughts compelling you to consume. What feelings (e.g. tension in my forehead) are you feeling in different parts of your body?

_____

_____

_____

_____

2. What do you feel is your inadequacy? Try and define your source of feelings of inadequacy as specifically as possible. Are they sourced in fear of something? What are your thoughts associated with this fear?

_____

_____

_____

_____

3. How do you feel consuming will help with this inadequacy?

_____

_____

_____

_____

4. Before you consume, ask yourself the following four questions:

E. Will it bring me power of the genuine [internally authentic] sort?

F. Will it increase my level of enlightenment?

G. Will it make me more whole?

H. Will it make me more loving?

15. Now notice with your senses what your body wants. If your connections feel tired, it could be sleep. If your throat is dry, it could be water. If you have pressure in your bladder or your bowels, maybe you want to go to the toilet. Write it down here:

_____

16. Is what you wrote down in step 6 different to what your mind wants you to consume? The secret to releasing yourself from excess is to start living from what you notice you want rather than what your mind says you should want.

_____

_____

17. Now go back and repeat step 2. Focus on the physical sensations you are having that your mind is associating with the compulsion to consume. Rate your level of pain or discomfort of not giving into the compulsion to consume on a level of 1-10 with 10 being intolerable agony and preferring to die.

_____

18. Reality test your pain/discomfort. Can you live with it? Can you survive it?

_____

19. Allow yourself to fully experience and notice those sensations now. The more you allow yourself to experience them, the more they will have been experienced fully and therefore disappear of their own accord. The alternative, which is resisting those sensations, allows those sensations to persist. The only way to ease them is to allow yourself to experience each physical sensation individually and to stop resisting its perceived unpleasantness. Your mind is a drama queen. The sensations are never as bad as you think they are. It helps if you notice when each sensation appears in your body and if you describe each sensation individually. Describe each sensation below now and then focus your attention on each in turn. Allow yourself to fully experience (and feel) each sensation.

_____

_____

_____

_____

_____

Chapter 7, Day 22: PART I, exercising awareness with doing - the conscious veto

Exercise for clearing your mind of distraction and moderating what gets into your to-do list. The more things you feel you should and shouldn't do, the further and further behind your expectations of yourself you fall, the more you shit on yourself, and the more demoralized you feel.

Instructions
1. Look at your to do list if you have one (if not skip to step 3). Mark only those items that are an absolute necessity to you and your family staying alive with an 'N' for necessity. Mark the things you think you should do with an 'S' for SHIT. One of the Golden rules of the Five connections is that when you should on yourself, you shit on yourself. Shitting on yourself is fairly demoralizing. Mark those things you genuinely want to do with a 'W' for want.

2. Look at your list again. Choose some of the 'S' items to veto and cross them off your list. What remains is more of what you want or need to do.

3. Practice this for the next week: every time you have a thought to do something, ask yourself if it is something you want or need to do. If it isn't, veto it. If you can notice the origin of the thought —what previous thoughts caused you to have that thought? Be aware that you are noticing yourself having the thought to do whatever it is, and you are consciously choosing to veto it.

PART II (from a Harvard Health Report on Positive Psychology)

To keep the burden of choice from robbing you of pleasure, go on a choice diet. For choices of no great consequence, limit the amount of time or number of options you'll consider. Cut off your opportunities for second guessing: stop looking at car or employment ads after you've made a commitment; go ahead and wrap or mail that gift; wear and launder your new pants so they can't be returned. When critical medical or financial choices need to be made, that's the time to put your Maximizer tendencies to work. But for the many small choices you make each day, try to narrow your choices quickly and make your decisions confidently.

Chapter 7, Day 23: Exercising awareness of time and money
PART I

Exercise for identifying what is enough when it comes to work and to money

Instructions

1. How many hours of work would you like to accomplish in a working week? **Tip**: if it's over 40 you may have a problem

_____

7. What do you consider to be enough hours for you to work a week?

_____

8. How many activities would you like to accomplish in a week in addition to your work?

9. How many hours would a week do you want to spend on those activities?

10. How much money do you want to earn as a minimum in a working week?

11. What do you consider enough money for you to earn in a working week? **Tip**: once you cover basic needs (estimated at $40000 USD a year in the USA) any increase in your cash levels will not have an impact on your happiness

PART II

For whenever you feel dominated by thoughts of money or all the things you still have to do at work. This also works as a relaxation and grounding-in-the-present-moment technique for any scenario.

12. Become conscious of the feeling of the air going in and out of your body as you breathe.

13. How many seconds do you pause between the end of the in breath and the beginning of the out breath?

14. How many seconds do you pause between the end of the out breath and the beginning of the in breath?

15. Repeat the above for at least three breaths

Chapter 7, Day 24: Exercising awareness of desire - the tempting way to self control

Exercise for when you feel compelled to do something you know isn't healthy for your relationships, nor for your authentic being, nor your Five connections.

Instructions:
The next time you feel a compulsive desire to cheat on a partner you love, take a time out for your being and do the following.

6. Accept that you are attracted to other people than your partner. If the other person is flirting with you or making physical (sexual) advances towards you, tell them the following, in your own words.

   I accept I am attracted to you, AND, I also accept that I am in a relationship with someone I love so as long as I am in that relationship I want to respect that love.

7. Notice the sensations in your body associated with your feelings compelling you to cheat. What feelings (e.g. tension) are you feeling in different parts of your body?

   _____

   _____

   _____

   _____

   _____

8. What do you feel is your inadequacy? Try and define your source of feelings of inadequacy as specifically as possible. Are they sourced in a feeling that you are not getting enough attention/affection from your current partner? Is it that you don't feel you can communicate fully with your partner? When was the last time YOU initiated an open and honest conversation with your partner?

   _____

_____

_____

_____

9. How do you feel cheating on your partner will help with this inadequacy?

_____

_____

_____

_____

10. Before you cheat, ask yourself the following four questions:

    a. Will it bring me power of the genuine [internally authentic] sort?

    b. Will it increase my level of enlightenment?

    c. Will it make me more whole?

    d. Will it make me more loving?

11. Now notice with your senses what your body wants. If your connections feel tired, it could be sleep. If your throat is dry, it could be water. If you have pressure in your bladder or your bowels, maybe you want to go to the toilet. Write it down here:

_____

_____

_____

The secret to being faithful to the one you love is that you start living from what you notice you want rather than what your mind says you should want, and you honestly communicate what you notice you want to the one you love.

Exercising awareness with conformity and moralizing how to stop shitting on yourself

Exercise for recognizing your shoulds and should nots, to minimize how much you shit on yourself. Every should and should not you attach importance to, demoralizes you. Every should and should not is about as good for your Happiness Animal's health as taking a shit on yourself before you go out the door.

Instructions

1. At home practice replacing the word 'toilet' with the word 'should' – even put a sign on the toilet door that says should.

2. On your phone or in a notepad, start a 'should shit log' for the next week starting right now. Every time you notice yourself saying the word 'should' write down 'I shit on myself' with the time and date.

3. What are your favorite limiting beliefs that your self imposes on your existence? (e.g. I don't know enough about this, I don't have time.) Write them down below.

_____

_____

_____

_____

_____

4. For every limiting belief you notice yourself saying over the next week, write down 'I squirt on myself' in your 'should shit log'.

5. Write down how you normally shoot yourself in the foot. (E.g. by making excuses, prioritizing something financial over something you want to do, or by getting distracted.)

_____

_____

_____

_____

Every time you notice yourself shooting yourself in the foot, write 'I constipate myself' in your 'should shit log'.

6. After a week of entries, re-read your 'should shit log'. Congratulations you have now identified the bullshit of your ego existence. Now flush it down the toilet.

For Happiness Coaching & Personal Training for Happiness visit:
www.happinessanimal.com or email the author:
w@happinessanimal.com
Please send your happiness postcards to the Facebook page
Facebook.com/TheHappinessAnimal or email the author.

71275124R00073

Made in the USA
Middletown, DE
21 April 2018